FDR Unmasked
73 Years of Medical Cover-ups
That Rewrote History

Steven Lomazow, M.D.

Oh, what a tangled web we weave, when first we practice to deceive.
Sir Walter Scott, 1806, Marmion, Canto Sixth, Stanza 17

Revised edition

ISBN
978-90-6299-326-0

Published by
Kugler Publications
P.O. Box 20538
1001 NM Amsterdam, The Netherlands
www.kuglerpublications.com

For my beloved wife, Suze Bienaimee

■ Table of Contents

■ About the author

Steven Lomazow M.D. is a board-certified neurologist in practice for 43 years. His first FDR biography, *FDR's Deadly Secret*, written with journalist Eric Fettmann, was published in 2010 by Public Affairs. He has written numerous scholarly articles for peer-reviewed medical journals, including "The Epilepsy of Franklin Delano Roosevelt" in *Neurology* in 2011. He is a reviewer for the Journal of Medical Biography.

Dr. Lomazow has served as a trustee of the FDR Library and Museum at Hyde Park, New York and as president of the Medical History Society of New Jersey. He is the current President of the Neurological Association of New Jersey.

■ Acknowledgments

Above all, I must thank my beloved wife, Suze Bienaimee, who understands more than anyone else how important this project is to me and who has been supportive beyond belief.

My involvement with FDR began 15 years ago with preparations for "FDR's Deadly Secret" with coauthor journalist Eric Fettmann, then an associate editorial editor for Rupert Murdoch's *New York Post*. Finding a literary agent and, subsequently, a publisher was surprisingly easy. In retrospect, Eric did all the heavy lifting through his connections in the publishing world. He was also a gifted and experienced writer. Without him, the project would never have gotten off the ground.

The book provided me with an introduction to the wonderful staff of the FDR Library, originally as a researcher and then as a trustee owing to the kindness of then director Lynn Bassanese. Archivists Kirsten Carter, Herman Eberhardt, and Bob Clark; programs director Cliff Laube; and Lynn's successor Paul Sparrow have been extraordinarily kind and generous with their time and friendship. Thanks also and congratulations to always amiable and welcoming new director, Bill Harris.

FDR has also brought me some of my closest friendships, including Dr. Hal "Toby" Raper, of Atlanta, who grew up in Warm Springs, and his lovely wife, Kathy, and Kathryn Smith of Anderson, South Carolina, and her husband, Leo, through her relationship with Missy LeHand's grandnieces and her book *The Gatekeeper*. They are both devoted FDR scholars and have been tremendously supportive of this project. Kathryn kindly volunteered to take on the tedious yet critically important project of indexing this book. And, of course, my wonderfully ebullient friend Jan Kenneth Herman, a fellow Long Islander and former Navy medical historian who interviewed Howard Bruenn and soon came to learn firsthand about historical deception. I will never forget our trips to the Cary Grayson archive in Staunton, Virginia, and my tour of the "old" Naval Hospital at Foggy Bottom, where the "moons of Mars" telescope is located.

Without the kindness and generosity of Bill Heiter, major portions of the story could never have been brought to light. To bring his father, Dr. Les Heiter, out of the shadows of history has been an unimpeachable and glorious historical revelation.

Having only written medical papers previously, this book literally forced me to learn how to write. Writers of dozens of books, Tom and Dorothy Hoobler provided their expertise and research. Michael Dolan, editor of *American History Magazine*, provided editing suggestions but, more than anyone else, taught me the nuts and bolts of writing, from the "Oxford comma" down to the basics of punctuation, sentence structure, and style. Without "Dolan 101," this book would have been a grammatical disaster.

Another major cog in the wheel was Deborah Gardner, historian/curator of Roosevelt House in NYC. Deborah went over the manuscript word by word on two separate occasions and provided invaluable fact and content checking, most importantly with respect to Eleanor Roosevelt. Her knowledge of the Roosevelts is unsurpassed. My thanks also for the kindness and support of the director of Roosevelt House, Harold Holzer.

Many physicians have reinforced my belief as to the credibility of what I have been writing, including my friend and the world's expert on lupus erythematosus, rheumatologist par excellence Dr. Robert Lahita. I've always referred to "Dr. Bob" as the smartest physician I have ever met and still have no reason to doubt my assessment. The great Dr. Robert Ruben, aside from finding a publisher, has encouraged me from the start, as have other members of the Grolier Club in New York City, including world politics maven David A. Andelman, who has kindly provided the foreword; Dr. Andrew Nadell, of San Francisco, who has arranged my inaugural speaking gig; fellow magazine enthusiast Dr. Len Banco; book designer par excellence Jerry Kelly; and the ever enthusiastic Eve Kahn.

All along, I have been helped by William Villano, whom I first met when he began helping with cataloguing my magazine collection. Will did some stints at the FDR Library and has made himself the world's expert on Vincent Astor, an important part of the book. He is now an archivist at the National Holocaust Museum and has a very bright future. The depth of his knowledge never ceases to amaze me.

A list of acknowledgments would not be complete without some of my dearest and most supportive friends, the brilliant Larry Fox, Professor "Jimble," James Kimble, of Seton Hall University; my fellow zealot for "United We Stand"; Elwood Taylor; as well as the pulp magazine contingent, John Gunnison and

John Locke; and my confidante, dear friend, and long-time dealer in rare and collectible magazines, Richard Samuel West.

And, lastly, of course, thanks to Franklin and Eleanor Roosevelt, the most consequential couple in American history!

■ Foreword
■ Fatal Consequences

David A. Andelman

What are the consequences of the disability of the leader of a great nation at peace or even more dangerously at war? I have been in on any number of death watches throughout my career: Tito in Yugoslavia; Brezhnev, Andropov, Chernenko in the Soviet Union. Beyond the death watches—simply the question of the health of the leader, his (or her) ability to carry on the demanding, daily business of running a major nation—or even a small one. Recall, most immediately, when Donald Trump was rushed to Walter Reed Medical Center with COVID-19 as that pandemic was reaching its peak.

None of these episodes were pretty. Each of them sapped the vitality of the nation and the people they led. Merely the energy alone that went into the act of keeping secret the true nature of this disability consumed vast resources and diverted the attention of officials whose talents would have been so fruitfully employed in the betterment of their own nation and securing their place in the world.

In the case of Yugoslavia, maintaining in power Tito, the only glue that held together this disparate nation of republics fused in the crucible of the peace that ended World War I, was a gargantuan effort. A tribute to this futility was the speed in which each of these nation-states used the centrifugal forces unleashed by Tito's death to declare their independence and join respectively the United Nations, in most cases the European Union, and for some, NATO. From Tito's unitary empire sprang the nations of Croatia, Slovenia, Serbia, Montenegro, Macedonia, Bosnia-Herzegovina, and eventually Kosovo. Most are fully functioning, western-styled democracies, some with admirable prosperity, all with a determination to pursue an independent course—with the absence at their collective head of a leader who was little more than a feudal warlord. Tito had effectively been placed and maintained there by democracies that thought only of their individual self-interests and the need to return a semblance of peace to this disparate, occasionally violent kaleidoscope of nationalities that clung to the southeastern fringes of Europe.

As for the Soviet leaders, they successively had a single goal—to maintain themselves and their colleagues in charge of perhaps the world's largest and longest-running kleptocracy. And each of them succeeded until the entire structure came suddenly crashing down around them.

Imagine, however, a nation and a leader who may have had the capacity to put a brake on that process or at the very least minimize its impact. But that leader, wracked with pain and illness, was unable either to recognize or react appropriately to the toxic sleight of hand that was being perpetrated by the Soviet leader of that time. And this leader—Franklin Delano Roosevelt—had been elected in an honorable fashion by perhaps the longest-running and most functional democracy. The problem faced by those who were closest to him was little different from the one faced by a succession of trusted advisers to generations of Soviet leaders through the twentieth century. America's leader was desperately, it turned out fatally ill. But he was unwilling to publicly acknowledge this pressing reality.

At their peak, of course, the leaders of the Allied nations battling Hitler were unparalleled in their ability to set a direction and goals that, while in some cases deeply malevolent, were achievable by the force and agility of their will.

By the end of World War II, as the victorious allies sought to shape and define the world that would emerge from its ashes, none of the Allied leaders was so endowed with unchallenged or unchallengeable power than Joseph Stalin. The problem was that the one individual in any position to restrain his ambitions was an American leader in profound pain and decline. Moreover, enormous efforts were being expended to make certain that no one would have any sense of the depths and dysfunction of this leader's capacities.

Franklin Roosevelt had been leading an entire civilization, the free world's pinnacle of democracy in an existential clash. Yet by the time we begin to draw toward the conclusion of this conflict, FDR was approaching the end of his rope. It is this drama that Steven Lomazow so admirably unpacks in this riveting volume. In this case, it would be worth examining the price we are paying today.

The price especially revolves around the Yalta Conference. Winston Churchill was at the peak of his powers. Joseph Stalin insisted that the conference be held at the Black Sea resort where he had for years maintained a retreat. His doctors held that he was too ill to travel, but in fact this was more likely attributable to Stalin's fear of flying. As for Roosevelt, he would die just two months later, though at the time he attempted to portray himself in full command of his facilities and his nation. As Dr. Lomazow details, that was far from the truth. Roosevelt was deeply ill, "encumbered by metabolic encephalopathy—'brain fog'—due to continuous pain, severe hypertension, multiple organ failure, and the side effects and interactions of the cocktail of drugs being used to treat those ailments." Roosevelt was incapable of standing up to Stalin and his most fundamental demands. "Encephalopathy diminishes the ability to maintain attention and multitask—a significant impairment for a man who prided himself as the hub of the wheel in every important matter of policy," Dr. Lomazow writes. Above all, Roosevelt was in the very midst of the complex negotiations with a Soviet dictator utterly in command of his material and his views of where he wanted to take the world. Roosevelt's failure to restrain Stalin's demands would change the course of the twentieth century and lay the basis for conflicts that have marked the twenty-first century as well.

Stalin came to Yalta with a sweeping collection of demands that would, he secretly believed, secure the position of Russia in post–World War II Europe and enable it to restore the powers that had been drained from it by years of an all-out war of survival. Since Roosevelt was focused on the need to lure the Soviet Union into turning to Japan and the defeat of the third Axis power once Germany and Italy had been crushed, the American president was incapable of fending off Stalin's leading demands—simply too ill to challenge the Soviet leader. Above all, he failed utterly to appreciate the consequences of giving in to Stalin, nor did his advisers appreciate how ill Roosevelt was—and the need to insulate him from the decision-making process at Yalta.

The particular demands of Stalin that Roosevelt failed to contest, indeed appeared to embrace simply and passively, stand out for their future impact on global affairs in particularly toxic fashion. Especially so were Stalin's demand for a Soviet veto in the United Nations Security Council and that all "democratic peoples" be the determinants of the future of East European governments—effectively a Soviet sphere of influence across the continent. Both had a major influence on the future course of history in Europe and far beyond—especially cementing the Soviet Union as one of the two superpowers for nearly a half century of communist power, throughout what would become the Cold War.

The Soviet Bloc

Stalin insisted that Poland, the avenue through which the Soviet Union and earlier the Russian Empire had been invaded on multiple occasions, needed a special status. While Allied forces were still battering Germany from the West, Soviet troops had already swept through and effectively seized control of Poland, installing a procommunist provisional government. So, with the long-standing Russian philosophy that in the end it was boots-on-the-ground that established undeniable authority—a concept that even in the twenty-first century Vladimir Putin embraced in a host of his adventures from Georgia to Crimea and onward to Ukraine—Stalin insisted Russia's interests in that nation be paramount. Roosevelt and especially Churchill believed that the noncommunist Polish government-in-exile that had spent the war based in London was most representative of the Polish people. In the end, Poland was sold out—the Yalta agreement simply declaring that a "more broadly based" government should be established in Poland pending free elections at some indeterminate future that never arrived. Any number of American officials were persuaded, with considerable reason, that this condemned Poland to a communist future.

But that was only the beginning for half of Europe that would be forced at gunpoint to bow to the will of Stalin and his Kremlin successors. Roosevelt had agreed that future governments of all nations bordering the Soviet Union would need to be "friendly" to Moscow. Indeed, it was at Yalta that Roosevelt's failure to draw a red line across Stalin's aspirations led at least nine nations into a half century of communist enslavement. Roosevelt and Churchill believed, retrospectively demonstrating unparalleled naivete, that by accepting Stalin's "pledge" to allow representatives into Warsaw's provisional government in preparation for free elections, they had done all that was possible to guarantee a democratic future for this nation. Poland had become Hitler's first victim after Britain's Neville Chamberlain sold them out at Munich for a scrap of paper he proclaimed represented "peace in our time." Now, at Yalta, Poland would be sold out one more time.

Poland was joined by at least five other European nations who had been conquered by Hitler, which at Yalta would wind up being enslaved yet again. Bowing to Stalin's demands and banking on his "promise" to allow free elections in all of Eastern Europe liberated from Nazi occupation, including Czechoslovakia, Hungary, Bulgaria, and Romania, Roosevelt and Churchill agreed that all future governments bordering the Soviet Union should be "friendly" to the Kremlin. Stalin wanted a buffer zone of his "near abroad" that would pledge fealty to him and his successors—a loyalty that would at least twice in the next quarter century be guaranteed by Soviet armor and military might. As the Allies gathered at Yalta, Soviet troops were on the ground in Poland and advancing rapidly through the rest of Nazi-controlled eastern and central Europe. Moreover, with Roosevelt clearly marshaling his limited strength for other battles, the American leader had little choice but to agree to Stalin's demands. The consequences of such an agreement that effectively embraced, as well, Stalin's philosophy of governance and dominance became increasingly clear as the Cold War developed and as NATO faced off with the Warsaw Pact. Twice—in 1956 in Hungary and again in 1968 in Czechoslovakia—Soviet-bloc forces intervened to put a halt to movements that threatened to weaken the iron control the Kremlin exerted in each of its "satellite" nations. Even after communism was itself dismantled in the last years of the twentieth century, this same DNA of Stalinism would continue to define the nature of Russian behavior into the twenty-first century as well.

The United Nations and Stalin's Veto

A veto was the final nail in the coffin of Roosevelt's dream of a United Nations that Stalin saw instead as simply another tool in the Kremlin's toolbox. As it turns out, it may have been the most potent, certainly the most lasting—enduring well past the Communist experiment itself. It was the one outcome of Yalta that would have implications ranging far beyond the structure of Europe east and west. Indeed, it would prove indispensable to generations of tyrants and demagogues of all stripes. At Yalta, Stalin was prepared to entertain a United Nations, even a Security Council, along the lines that Roosevelt was advocating. What he did not want was a Security Council that was in a position to launch military activities against any Soviet actions where he felt his desires were justified or appropriate. Accordingly, Stalin demanded and got a veto as one of five "permanent members" of the Security Council. And that made all the difference in any number of toxic moments where the Soviet Union had any stakes that countered the interests or desires of the rest of the (free) world. It would prove useful, equally, to a succession of Chinese leaders and their sympathizers whose rise could hardly have been anticipated at the time by either Roosevelt or Churchill. Roosevelt, in his rare clear moments, might have anticipated the implications of this veto for America and the West, but he clearly did not foresee the vast abuses the veto could spawn. Or perhaps he was simply in no position to counter Stalin's demand.

The extent of the abuse of the veto power, especially by Russia, is truly stunning. Since February 16, 1946, when the Soviet Union cast the first veto on a draft resolution regarding the withdrawal of foreign troops from Lebanon and Syria, the veto has been invoked 293 times. The imbalance is especially striking. Russia and the Soviet Union have cast a total of 120 vetoes, nearly half of all. The United States did not cast the first of its 82 vetoes until March 17, 1970. Britain and France have not cast a single veto since December 1989. Since the end of the Cold War and in recent years, the pace of the veto's use has only quickened. Since 2011 through December 2020, Russia cast 19 vetoes, 14 of which dealt with Syria. Eight of the nine Chinese vetoes in this period were over Syria and one dealt with Venezuela. Still, the threat of the veto alone has prevented any number of questions from even being brought before the Security Council. Today, most such measures that do reach a vote—and a veto—are made purely for symbolic purposes, to demonstrate graphically the stakes of the permanent members of the Council in an issue.

The Aftermath

It did not take long for the West to recognize how much had been lost at Yalta. Roosevelt himself, of course, lived to see none of these consequences. As Dr. Lomazow documents, he died barely two months after returning from Yalta. By March 1945, it was quite clear that Stalin had no intention of respecting his vague promises of political freedom in Poland or indeed any other of his near-abroad neighbors. Soviet troops quickly crushed a pro-western provisional government in Lublin, Poland, in preparations for sham elections in 1945 that would set a pattern throughout the Cold War and indeed through to Crimea, the Donbas and southern Ukraine in the twenty-first century. Harry Truman, Roosevelt's successor, would prove more skeptical of Stalin and his pledges, but by the time these leaders met at Potsdam in July 1945 to cement the final terms for the armistice, Stalin's forces had already occupied virtually the entire eastern half of the continent.

There remains, of course, the open question of whether Stalin could ever have been thwarted in his demands short of dispensing with the Soviet Union refusing to enter the war against Japan (which the Soviets did only at the very last moment, nearly four months after Roosevelt's death, and with little change to the ultimate direction of hostilities). At the same time, there was also the risking of an all-out conflict in Europe with weakened but hardly neutralized Soviet forces that the American people had little or no appetite to engage with at that moment.

By March 1946, barely a year after Yalta, Stalin's gains were so clearly defined that Churchill hardly hesitated to proclaim in his memorable address at Westminster College: "From Stettin in the Baltic to Trieste in the Adriatic, an Iron Curtain has descended across the continent."

In so many respects, this was Churchill's and FDR's most lasting global legacy.

■ Preface

FDR Unmasked chronicles Franklin Delano Roosevelt's life from a physician's perspective. It tells a harrowing story of heroic achievement by a great leader determined to impart his vision of freedom and democracy to the world while under constant siege by serious medical problems.

Time magazine wrote on June 10, 1940, "The mystery. Last week, Franklin Delano Roosevelt, 58 years old, seven generations removed from a Dutch settler of 1644, son of a country gentleman and the belle of the Hudson River valley, was head of the last great democracy still at peace, with 33 weeks left of his second term. Yet, although he was in his eighth year as President, although he had moved, worked, eaten, laughed, exhorted, prayed in the intensest glare of public scrutiny, although his every facial grimace, the tone of his voice, each mannerism, *the dark mole over his left eyebrow*, the mole on his right cheek— although all these were public property, intimate to every U.S. citizen, still there was no man in the U.S. who could answer the question, Who Is Franklin Roosevelt?" This gross lack of understanding is not accidental, but rather the result of a series of cover-ups that began in 1921 and actively persisted until 1994. *FDR Unmasked* takes on the enigma of FDR by categorically exposing well-entrenched, utterly false narratives.

It has been nearly eighty years since FDR died, yet large portions of his life remain a mystery. Conventional belief holds that after triumphing over a mid-career bout with polio, he went on to serve two vigorous terms as governor of New York and three-plus more as president of the United States, succumbing unexpectedly to a stroke on April 12, 1945. In truth, Franklin spent those eventful twenty-four years battling swarms of maladies including polio's ongoing crippling effects, life-threatening gastrointestinal bleeding, two incurable cancers, severe cardiovascular disease, and epilepsy.

From the onset of polio in 1921 until his death, Franklin, his family, his inner circle of advisers, and teams of physicians assiduously disguised the state of his health, promoting the fantasy of a robust leader who was always in excellent physical condition for a man his age. Severe heart disease was not admitted until twenty-five years after his death, and then only as part of a new and larger cover-up to conceal other severe medical problems. These deceptions still dominate the present-day narrative of Franklin's health, especially in his later years.

The postmortem cover-up was masterminded by his daughter, Anna Roosevelt Halsted, and her physician husband, working in concert with FDR's cardiologist, Dr. Howard Bruenn. They perpetrated this hoax by manufacturing a false medical narrative and publishing it in a prominent medical journal. This was designed to hoodwink historians, beginning with James MacGregor Burns in the late 1960s, who unwittingly and enthusiastically accepted the Halsted/Bruenn misrepresentations as fact and included them in his Pulitzer Prize-winning 1970 Roosevelt biography, *Soldier of Freedom*. Anna died in 1975, but Bruenn continued to promote and enhance the deception in interviews and films until shortly before his death at age 90 in 1995.

Independent of the Halsteds and Bruenn, Margaret "Daisy" Suckley, FDR's "closest companion" and confidante, carried out her own cover-up, keeping a detailed diary which she bowdlerized to exclude firsthand observations of his most serious medical problems, then left it under her bed. The diary was found after her death in 1991. In addition, Suckley was archivist at the FDR Library from its opening in June 1941 until 1963 and had control of its contents.

Another piece of the puzzle was uncovered in 2016 when an unusually thick file was found at the FDR Library related to a "vacation" cruise FDR took over Easter 1934. The file was dense with documents that included a telegram addressed to President Roosevelt from a cancer radiation specialist as well as urgent encoded communications between White House press secretaries and the yacht's owner, Vincent Astor, Roosevelt's longtime friend and relative by marriage. The cruise was unexpectedly extended and important events in the president's schedule were postponed after FDR became seriously ill from the medical treatment he had secretly received.

The documents also revealed that a previously unknown physician, Dr. W. Leslie Heiter, had been aboard Astor's yacht with the President. Further research into the mystery doctor struck gold. Fortunately for history, his son, Bill, had preserved and curated his father's papers. Aside from showing that Dr. Heiter had trained as a cancer surgeon in New York City, this previously unknown archive traced his association with FDR back to his days as Governor of New York. *FDR Unmasked* reveals the important story of Dr. Heiter's relationship with Governor/President Roosevelt, both as his patient and his friend.

FDR Unmasked is first to present convincing evidence of Roosevelt's battle with prostate cancer, underpinned by FBI memoranda, reliable firsthand information from multiple physicians interviewed by medical sleuth Dr. Harry Goldsmith, the Suckley diary, and even a shocking admission by Eleanor Roosevelt to actress Veronica Lake that her husband was being treated for the disease. As with the other important medical aspects of Roosevelt's health, the book includes an explanation of the history, diagnosis, and contemporary treatment of prostate cancer, targeted to a lay audience.

Yet another new and groundbreaking story in *FDR Unmasked* is his highly consequential friendship with Vincent Astor, the closest with any man in his adult life. To truly understand the "real" Franklin Delano Roosevelt, the one behind his mask of deception, it is important to understand their almost brotherly relationship.

FDR has been labeled a "Traitor to his Class." This may have been so for his politics, but not for his closely guarded private life. *FDR Unmasked* reveals the truth of his inner workings. His early life is presented to provide readers with the greatest possible understanding of the roots of his charismatic yet ever-deceptive personality.

Researching this book has been a voyage of discovery and it is a privilege to present an unexpurgated medical biography of the most consequential American of the twentieth century.

■ Chapter 1
■ A Star Is Born

Franklin Delano Roosevelt's first health crisis occurred on the day he was born. His parents, James and Sara, were expecting their first child at Springwood, their Hyde Park, New York, estate. The baby was overdue. A nurse had been on duty for two weeks before Sara went into labor at 7:30 p.m. on a snowy Sunday, January 29, 1882. She struggled through the night. At 7:30 a.m., Mr. James, as he was known, summoned Dr. Edward H. Parker, five miles away in Poughkeepsie. The doctor arrived at 9:30 a.m.

Monday passed with Sara's cries of pain becoming more desperate. Dr. Parker came downstairs only long enough to inform Mr. James of his grave concern for the lives of mother and child. To save Sara's life, Parker administered chloroform, a general anesthetic introduced in 1847 in Britain.[1] American physicians had been leery of the drug—which posed a risk for mothers-to-be and newborn babies due to respiratory depression.[2]

Sara drifted into peaceful unconsciousness. Her son, weighing a full ten pounds, emerged silent with blue-tinged skin. Dr. Parker blew air into his lungs and the newborn let out a reassuring cry. "I was given too much chloroform, and it was nearly fatal to us both," Sara later wrote. "The nurse said she never expected the baby to be alive."[3]

---

1 The first demonstration of the anesthetic use of chloroform in humans was by Scottish obstetrician James Y. Simpson in 1847. Chloroform was used during the birth of Queen Victoria's eighth and ninth children in 1853 and 1857.
2 America's most influential gynecologist, J. Marion Sims, preferred the use of diethyl ether, which was first publicly demonstrated at the Massachusetts General Hospital by dentist William T. Morton on October 16, 1846. Sims later made it public that his fellow southerner, Crawford Long, had been using the anesthetic in Georgia since the early 1840s. Long is now credited with discovering its use.
3 Roosevelt, S.D., *My Boy Franklin: As Told by Mrs. James Roosevelt to Isabel Leighton and Gabrielle Forbush.* New York: Ray Long & Richard R. Smith, 1933, 12.

Franklin's difficult birth was the first of many health challenges in a sixty-three-year life punctuated by illness. According to one throat specialist, he faced "a lifetime series of sieges of the common cold, sinusitis, pharyngitis, tonsillitis, laryngitis, tracheitis, bronchitis, influenza, and pneumonia,"[4] and those were just the maladies that involved his respiratory tract.

Even the boy's name was a consequence of a health tragedy. For generations, Roosevelts had alternated the names of firstborn males between James and Isaac, but Sara was determined to name her son after her father, Warren Delano, Jr. Sara prevailed over Roosevelt tradition, but there was another consideration she could not overcome. Her brother Warren Delano III's four-year-old namesake had recently died of typhoid fever and he asked that the newborn not bear the name.

So it was that the only child of James and Sara was christened Franklin Delano Roosevelt on March 20, 1882, at St. James Episcopal Church in Hyde Park, New York. The boy was named for Sara's uncle Franklin Delano, who had a childless marriage with Laura Astor, granddaughter of John Jacob Astor, the richest man in America.[5] One of Franklin's two godfathers was Elliott Roosevelt, a scion of the branch of the family that resided on Long Island.

The James/Isaac succession ended with Franklin's father. After graduation from Harvard Law School, Mr. James amassed a small fortune in coal and railroads and joined the Whig Party. He became a Democrat when the Whigs disintegrated over slavery. The Oyster Bay Roosevelts were abolitionists and joined the Republican party of Abraham Lincoln.

Franklin's parents were brought together by another health tragedy. In 1854, James, twenty-five, married Rebecca Howland, who bore them a son christened with the odd name of James Roosevelt Roosevelt,[6] known as "Rosy."[7] After Mr. James's and Rebecca's home burned down in 1866, he purchased a house he renamed Springwood, on a six-hundred-acre estate in the Dutchess County town of Hyde Park, for $40,000 ($1,400,000 in 2022).

---

4 Fabricant, N., "Franklin D. Roosevelt's Nose and Throat Ailments." *Eye, Ear, Nose and Throat Monthly*, February, 1957.

5 The name suited him well. FDR identified with his Delano heritage as much or more than he did with the Roosevelt side.

6 Mr. James did not wish his first son to be burdened as a "Junior."

7 Rosy was six months older than his step-mother, Sara. He married into the Astor family in 1880.

Rebecca's heart began to fail in 1875 and she died in August 1876.[8] Emerging from mourning, James sought to remarry. After his cousin Anna "Bamie" Roosevelt politely rejected him,[9] her mother made introductions to Sara Delano. James was smitten. Tall and beautiful, the twenty-six-year-old Sara was concerned about becoming an old maid.[10] James was twice her age, but that did not seem to matter since he reminded her in the best ways of her father. Warren Delano Jr. knew Mr. James by reputation. "James Roosevelt is the first person who has made me realize that a Democrat can be a gentleman," he said.[11,12]

Sara's father had made his fortune in the "China trade," illegally importing Indian-grown opium to the Celestial Kingdom, a profession his grandson later referred to with a smile, telling White House visitors that his grandfather had been a drug smuggler. Delano lost his fortune in the Panic of 1857, returned to China in 1860, and amassed an even larger one. He reunited with his family in China in 1862. They returned to America three years later. "The Delanos were the first people I met who were able to do what they wanted to do without wondering where to obtain the money," Franklin's wife Eleanor later recalled.[13]

James and Sara were married in October 1880 at Algonac, the Delano estate near Newburgh, New York, on the west bank of the Hudson River. The new-lyweds left that November for a honeymoon in Europe. By the time they returned the following September, Sara was pregnant.

Because of Franklin's difficult birth, doctors cautioned Sara against another pregnancy. The years from 1884 to 1887 are absent from her journal. Scholars[14] have speculated that Sara destroyed the pages to protect the privacy of her marital relations, as her only defense against another pregnancy was abstinence.[15]

8 Smith, J.E., *FDR*. New York: Random House, 2007, 326.
9 Anna "Bamie" Roosevelt was TR's older sister. Martha Bulloch "Mittie" Roosevelt was Eleanor's grandmother.
10 Smith, J.E., 15.
11 Brands, H.W., *Traitor to His Class. New York:* Anchor Books, 2009, 6.
12 *Ibid.*
13 Roosevelt, E., *Autobiography of Eleanor Roosevelt*. New York: Harper & Brothers, 1961, 47 as cited in Smith, J.E., 639, 22*n*.
14 Smith, J.E., 642, 13*n*.
15 *Ibid.*

Franklin spent his first fourteen years tended to by governesses, nurses, and tutors. Sara breast-fed him for nearly a year and bathed him until he was eight. She saved his letters, along with most of his toys and clothing. Her diary records his every action. He could read and write by age five and was also tutored in French and German. His earliest surviving letter involved health matters. "I am very sorry you have a cold and are in bed," he wrote his mother. "I hope by tomorrow you will be able to be up. I am glad to say that my cold is better.... Your loving Franklin D. Roosevelt."[16]

Hardly a moment of young Franklin's day went unscheduled. He was awakened at seven, breakfasted at eight and tutored until eleven. Lunch was at noon, followed by more lessons until four. Two hours were allotted for play. Dinner was at six and bedtime at eight. Sara's control extended to the children she permitted to visit Springwood—never overnight and not too often during the day, she insisted.

By the time he was four, Franklin was accompanying his father on a pony for daily inspection tours of Springwood. "Franklin never knew what it meant to have the kind of respect for his father that is composed of equal parts of awe and fear," Sara wrote. "The regard in which he held him, amounting to worship, grew out of a companionship ... and his father's never-failing understanding of the little problems that seem so grave to the child who is faced with them. His father never laughed at him.... They were such a gay pair when they went off on long rides together."[17] Mr. James took his five-year-old son to meet his friend, fellow Democrat President Grover Cleveland, during a family trip to Washington, D.C. "My little man, I am making a strange wish for you," the president told his visitor. "It is that you may never be President of the United States."[18]

Mr. James often took his son aboard his fifty-one-foot sailboat, the *Half-Moon*. The boy learned to handle it as soon as he was tall enough to see over the wheel. By sixteen, Franklin was commanding his own sloop, the *New Moon*, and navigating the tides at the family's Canadian summer retreat on Campobello Island, located on the Bay of Fundy just off the coast of Maine.[19]

16 Roosevelt, E. ed., *F.D.R. His Personal Letters, Early Years.* New York: Duell, Sloan & Pearce, 1947, 206.
17 Roosevelt, S.D., 120.
18 Smith, J.E., 23.
19 Beschloss, M., "Sailing Was More Than Respite for Roosevelt and Kennedy." New York Times, September 15, 2015.

Young Franklin's cloistered homes at Hyde Park and Campobello were his universe. He entertained himself by escaping into worlds in which he was the only inhabitant. Avocations played an important role throughout his life. Before he was ten, he was shooting and collecting birds, and gathered examples of over 300 species. His birding diary, compiled over three-and-a-half years, contained seventy-nine pages of sightings. For his eleventh birthday, he read his treatise on "Birds of the Hudson Valley" to his assembled family. Sara's father was so impressed he presented his grandson with life membership in New York's American Museum of Natural History. Franklin often referred to the event as the greatest thrill of his early life.[20] He also took over his mother's stamp collection, an interest he pursued with enthusiasm until literally the day he died. On the other hand, family stories about his nineteen-year-old aunt Laura Delano's slow, agonizing death in 1884 after being burned triggered a lifelong fear of fire.[21]

Sara and James taught their son to respond to adversity by keeping a stiff upper lip. He used his mettle for the remainder of his life. Franklin's resistance to his mother's meddling tempered him to be able to deal with adversity. "Certainly [Sara] would have dominated him if she could have done so, but Father ... was tough enough to resist her. His son James later wrote ... Indeed, I feel she strengthened his character by increasing his capacity for resistance."[22] As Franklin's daughter later noted: "Granny was a martinet, but she gave father the assurance he needed to prevail over adversity. Seldom has a young child been more constantly attended and incessantly approved by his mother."[23]

Franklin's active participation as a congregant and vestryman at St. James Episcopal Church of Hyde Park exerted a lifelong influence. "I always felt that my grandfather was a deeply religious person. And yet his profound sense of God was never ostentatious." said his oldest grandson, Curtis Roosevelt.[24]

His most serious childhood illness occurred in August 1888 at age six, when he contracted typhoid fever on an ocean liner bound for Liverpool. This highly infectious and often deadly disease is caused by ingesting water contaminated

---

20 Smith, J.E., 24.
21 An oil lamp spilled and ignited Laura's nightgown.
22 Roosevelt, J., Shalett, S., *Affectionately, F.D.R.* New York: Harcourt Brace, 1959, 25.
23 Smith, J.E., 25, as quoted in *The F.D.R. Memoirs.* New York: Doubleday, 1973, 24.
24 https://hydeparkhistorian.tumblr.com/post/171320294056/fdr-frustrated-clergyman (last accessed December 6, 2022).

with *Salmonella* bacteria.[25] At the first port of call, Queenstown, Ireland,[26] the captain wired ahead to have his physician cousin and a nurse meet the ship at Liverpool, where a tender, courtesy of the White Star Line's owner, ferried the Roosevelts to shore.[27] Franklin convalesced at the doctor's home on a diet of cold, boiled milk and chicken broth. By November, he was able to tolerate solid food and resume traveling. Had he not had access to the finest medical care—on this instance and others—he might not have lived to become president.

The Roosevelt family dynamic changed drastically when Franklin was eight. Mr. James suffered a heart attack at age sixty-two and was never again the energetic figure his son had known. Heart disease was felt to be worsened by emotional stress, so Franklin and Sara internalized their problems in fear of upsetting him. As biographer Kenneth Davis notes, "joined to his optimistic faith and sustained by it was a rare physical courage, a rare ability to bear pain stoically." During a trip in the family's private railroad car, for instance, a steel curtain rod broke loose and opened a deep gash above the boy's left eye. Franklin insisted his father not see him until the gushing blood had stopped.[28]

A London specialist recommended Mr. James visit Bad Nauheim, Germany, where mineral springs said to be good for the heart had led to the establishment of a popular spa.[29] The family began making annual visits in the spring of 1891.[30] During their first visit, Franklin was enrolled in public school for six weeks, but not again on three subsequent trips. Nearly a year after Franklin's final excursion to Germany, Sara permitted her fourteen-year-old "prince" to leave her nest and start the next chapter of his life at a rigorous New England boarding school. Even then she confided to her journal, "It is hard to leave our darling boy."[31]

25 The long list of celebrities who died of the disease includes Alexander the Great, Franz Schubert, Wilbur Wright, Abigail Adams, and Stephen A. Douglas.
26 It is known today as the port of Cobh.
27 White Star's most notorious vessel was RMS *Titanic*.
28 Davis, K., *FDR The Beckoning of Destiny 1882-1928*. New York: Random House, 1993, 84.
29 Bad Neuheim translates literally in German to "healing waters."
30 Ward, G., *Before the Trumpet*. New York: Harper Collins, 1985, 146.
31 Burns, J.M., *The Lion and the Fox*. New York: Harcourt Brace, 1956, 10.

■ Chapter 2
■ A Privileged Young Man

Groton School for Boys opened in 1884. Its charismatic founder, the Reverend Endicott Peabody, attracted upper-class clientele by offering to "cultivate manly, Christian character, having regard to moral and physical as well as intellectual development." Peabody "believed in religion, character, athletics, and scholarship—roughly in that order."[1,2] Tuition was $500 a year (nearly $18,000 in 2022) when Franklin was enrolled, twice what the average American family had to live on.[3]

Students at Groton entered a spartan, regimented communal life. The course of study was equivalent to today's seventh through twelfth grades. Peabody accepted just twenty-seven beginning students each year. Franklin was fourteen and his classmates were in their third year when he arrived in September 1896.

One of Groton's pillars was athletics. Pride of place went to football, which, Peabody explained, "is of profound importance for the moral even more than for the physical development of the boys…. [They] need an opportunity to endure hardness and, if it may be, suffering."[4] Never having participated in any team sport, Franklin was a rank outsider. Groton fielded eight football teams and he was assigned to the second-worst. He was also a stranger to baseball and wound up on the very worst nine. When sinus trouble later plagued him, he attributed the condition to having broken his nose on the football field. Like many other of his recollections, the athletic injuries Franklin described were enhanced. Geoffrey C. Ward's two comprehensive studies of Franklin's early life list nearly two dozen instances of "exaggerations."[5] "A good story

---

1 Smith, J.E., 27.
2 Peabody was the son of a wealthy banker. He attended England's Cambridge University then entered the clergy. He established the first Episcopal church in the Arizona territory before returning to Massachusetts to marry his first cousin and find his calling as an educator.
3 *Ibid.*, 24.
4 Ward, *BTT*, 184.
5 Ward's two books, *Before the Trumpet* and *A First Class Temperament*, are impeccably researched and encyclopedic about Franklin's life until 1928.

was sometimes preferable to an accurate one," biographer Jean Edward Smith wrote.[6]

Home schooling had kept Franklin apace academically but not socially. "The easy charm and cordiality that so pleased his mother and delighted his parents' friends seemed artificial to many of his contemporaries."[7] All the while, he represented himself as infallible. "If he was not doing as well as he believed he should, others must be at fault. He could not be," Geoffrey Ward wrote. Letters to his parents are replete with rationalizations for his shortcomings.[8] Throughout his life, Franklin rarely, if ever, admitted being wrong.

At Groton, Franklin paid the price for fourteen years of isolation from other children. He contracted measles, mumps, flu, and frequent colds. In the spring of his junior year, he came down with whooping cough, a disease so prevalent that infected students were allowed to attend classes. The school doctor diagnosed a weak heart and recommended he avoid strenuous activity but Franklin shook off the advice, telling his parents he thought the diagnosis was incorrect.[9]

When America declared war on Spain in 1898, Franklin and two classmates supposedly made plans to run away and join the Navy—until all three contracted scarlet fever. The school tracked down his parents in Europe to inform them their son had inflamed kidneys, a common complication of that bacterial infection. Sara and James cut their trip short and found Franklin in an upstairs room at the school infirmary "very thin and very white but better."[10] Warned that close contact with Franklin might cause her to transmit the disease to her sickly spouse, Sara bent the rules. "Several times each day, I would climb a tall rickety ladder and by seating myself on the top managed to see into the room and talk with our small, convalescent scapegrace. He loved to see me appear over the window sill," Sara later told her granddaughter.[11]

Franklin left Groton inculcated with Peabody's axioms—"competition is healthy, success comes from effort, reward is based on performance, religious observance and moral probity are indispensable to a productive life."[12] He

---

6 Smith, J.E., 13.
7 Ward, *BTT*, 203.
8 *Ibid.*
9 Brands, 27.
10 *Ibid.*, 201.
11 Roosevelt and Shalett, 21.
12 Smith, J.E., 28.

maintained a lifelong relationship with Peabody, who presided at his marriage and provided spiritual guidance at his first three presidential inaugurations.

The sea-loving Franklin had his heart set on attending the United States Naval Academy, but his parents convinced him that someday he would be managing the family estate, a role better suited to a lawyer than a military professional. At Harvard, Franklin was returned to the luxury and privilege he had enjoyed as a child. He shared a posh four-room apartment with his closest friend Lathrop Brown, and dined in a Cambridge restaurant at a table reserved for Groton graduates. The Roosevelt name brought a flurry of social opportunities.

Mr. James, Rosy, and Rosy's son, Franklin's nephew James Roosevelt Roosevelt, Jr., known as Taddy, were all Harvardians. Looking ahead to law school, Franklin majored in history and government. Economics left him cold. "I took economics in college for four years and everything I was taught was wrong," he said.[13]

The campus was a Republican hotbed. Franklin joined the Harvard Republican Club and worked in 1904 to reelect William McKinley and, of course, the incumbent's running mate, Eleanor's Uncle Theodore Roosevelt, also a Harvard alumnus.[14] He got his first thrill of campaign life marching in a torchlight parade of Harvard and M.I.T. men. "We wore red caps & gowns & marched … into Boston & thro' all the principal streets, about 8 miles in all," he wrote his parents." The crowds to see it were huge all along the route & we were dead tired at the end."[15]

Mr. James's health declined that fall and he died in his New York City hotel apartment on December 8, 1900, with Sara, Franklin, and Rosy at his side. The bulk of his estate went to Sara. Two years earlier she had inherited about $1.3 million ($46,000,000 in 2022) from her father. James's will provided Rosy and Franklin each with an annual income of about $6,000 ($213,000 in 2022). Rosy had married into the Astor fortune in 1880 but Franklin remained dependent on Sara's generosity to maintain a very high standard of living. As a minor, he was subject to the will's stipulation that he come "under the supervision of his mother,"[16] which Sara interpreted literally, taking up residence in a Boston

---

13 Miller, N., *F.D.R.: An Intimate History*. New York: Doubleday, 1983, 32.
14 Theodore Roosevelt was added to the ticket after McKinley's competent and well-liked Vice-President, New Jerseyan Garret A. Hobart, died of heart disease in 1899.
15 *Ibid.*, 34.
16 *Ibid.*, 36.

apartment. Franklin hosted social gatherings there and many girls took notice of his mother's dominance over him. Some remarked that the initials "F.D." stood for "feather duster," a pejorative term for a weak-willed person.

Extended family ties landed Franklin an invitation to the social event of the season, the January 1902 coming-out party of President Roosevelt's daughter Alice. With characteristic acerbity, Alice later recalled her cousin as "a good little mother's boy whose friends were dull, who belonged to the minor clubs and who was never at the really gay parties."[17] Franklin had been blackballed from Porcellian, Harvard's most prestigious club, to which his father, his half-brother, and his distant cousin, Theodore, had belonged.[18] He never got over the snub. Eleanor heard him talk about it so often she later said it had given him "an inferiority complex."[19]

Franklin's greatest success at Harvard was as a journalist, beginning in his freshman year as a reporter for the student-run newspaper, the *Daily Crimson*. He received his degree after three years but applied for graduate school to spend a fourth as editor-in-chief. He also joined clubs devoted to Harvard's history, including the prestigious Hasty Pudding[20] and Alpha Delta Phi, known around Harvard as "The Fly," and became librarian for both. He began collecting naval memorabilia, including prints, histories, biographies, and ship models. An avid bibliophile and discriminating collector, his library, particularly strong in naval history grew to contain over 23,000 books, periodicals, and catalogs.[21]

After a monkish adolescence at Groton, Franklin discovered girls at Harvard. He soon learned that filial piety and romance could clash when Sara vetoed his plan to invite young men and women to spend a weekend at Springwood. During his freshman year, the name of fifteen-year-old Alice Sohier began appearing in his diary, disguised in a code he devised to counteract his mother's snooping. Alice's father was a former Republican state legislator and an enthusiastic yachtsman—just the sort who would approve of a young

---

17 Meacham, J., *Franklin and Winston*. New York: Random House, 2003, 9.
18 This was probably because Franklin's reputation had been poisoned by his rebellious, socially unacceptable nephew Taddy, who had preceded him to Harvard by two years and left the school in disgrace after one.
19 Ward, *BTT*, 236.
20 FDR is one of five presidents who have been members, the others being John Adams and his son John Quincy Adams, TR, and John F. Kennedy.
21 His collection contains over 2,500 volumes on the American Navy and seventy devoted to John Paul Jones alone!.

Harvardian. At a Sohier family gathering, Franklin declared that he might someday become president. "Who else thinks so?" an older relative asked sarcastically, prompting laughter.[22]

In the summer of 1902, Franklin brought two classmates to Campobello aboard *New Moon* and anchored near the Sohiers' vacation home on the way. He treated his romantic interest to "a good long sail."[23] Geoffrey C. Ward hypothesizes Franklin had told Alice of his wish to have a large family. Alice responded by saying she had been told she could never bear children owing to the small size of her internal organs. Years later, she came clean to a friend: "I did not wish to be a cow."[24] Alice married an insurance executive and had two children with him.

Franklin had known his fifth-cousin Anna Eleanor Roosevelt from family gatherings. She was called Eleanor because both her mother and grandmother were named Anna. Her father, Elliott, Theodore's brother and Franklin's godfather, was a hopeless alcoholic for whom his only daughter never wavered in her reverence. On one occasion, Elliott took his young daughter for an outing in New York City and stopped at his gentleman's club, ostensibly for a short visit, instructing her to wait with the doorman. Six hours later he was carried out dead drunk.

Eleanor later recalled that her frequently absent father "rarely sent word before he arrived, but never was he in the house ... that I did not hear his voice the minute he entered the front door. Walking down stairs was far too slow. I slid down the banisters and usually catapulted into his arms before his hat was hung up," she wrote. "He dominated my life as long as he lived and was the love of my life for many years after he died."[25,26]

Eleanor's mother, Anna Hall, was a renowned beauty to whom her only daughter compared herself unfavorably, a habit her mother did little to discourage, deriding her with the nickname "Granny." A mild curvature of the spine required Eleanor to wear an uncomfortable steel brace for two years. Almost

---

22 *Ibid.*, 253.
23 *Ibid.*, 254.
24 *Ibid.*
25 Late in his 34-year life, Elliott lived in an alcohol sanitarium in Virginia and made sporadic visits to New York. He also fathered a child with a servant, Katherine, born in 1891. Elliott Roosevelt Mann worked as a bank auditor and died in 1977. Elliott died of a seizure after a failed suicide attempt.
26 Brands, 35.

six feet tall, she tended to stoop to appear more petite. Her unhappy home life brought about tension headaches and a recurring sense of impending dread.

Eleanor was orphaned at age nine, along with her younger brother; a second brother died in 1893. Her mother had died of diphtheria when she was eight and her absentee father passed away from chronic alcoholism less than two years later. She wound up living with her maternal grandmother, Mary Livingston Ludlow Hall, two alcoholic uncles, and a flighty aunt at her grandmother's Columbia County estate, Oak Terrace at Tivoli, and her New York City apartment.[27,28] One of Grandma Hall's few kindnesses was to send her fifteen-year-old interloper to Allenswood, a private school for girls in the Wandsworth borough of London. Eleanor's Aunt Bamie, affectionately known as "Auntie Bye," had attended the facility's previous incarnation in Paris and recommended the placement to relieve her niece from her toxic home environment.[29]

Allenswood's founder and headmistress, Mademoiselle Marie Souvestre, was witty and intellectually stimulating and became the compassionate older female figure Eleanor had never known. She taught her American student to dress and do her hair attractively, but most importantly fostered a sorely needed self-confidence.

The headmistress instilled progressive ideas and social consciousness in her students—teaching them about the union movement, the antisemitism of the Dreyfus affair in France, and Britain's use of concentration camps to imprison South Africans during the Boer War. While Eleanor was taken aback by her mentor's blatant atheism, she later called her three years in England "the happiest of my life" and returned home a transformed woman.[30] Souvestre was openly lesbian. Her relationship with her student was not at all sexual, though it probably exerted an influence upon the impressionable young American to adopt a more accepting view of same-sex relationships. Eleanor kept Souvestre's picture on her desk for the remainder of her life.

Soon after Eleanor's return to America, Franklin spotted her on a train and brought her to say hello to Sara, whose style and beauty reminded her of her

---

27 Oak Terrace at Tivoli was located on the east bank of the Hudson River.
28 Caroli, B.B., *The Roosevelt Women*. New York: Basic Books, 1998, 255–256.
29 At Tivoli, she was living with two drunken uncles and a vain flighty Aunt Pussie. Caroli, 255–256.
30 Ward, *BTT*, 296.

own mother's. The couple socialized throughout the summer of 1902. That winter, Theodore invited his niece to spend the New Year's holiday at the White House,[31] where she was reunited with Franklin, who had joined relatives to celebrate the holiday in Washington.

Franklin invited Eleanor to Hyde Park later that month for his twenty-first birthday party. They continued seeing each other until he went off to Europe with a Harvard friend. Upon his return, she came to Campobello, where Franklin took her on chaperoned sails aboard *Half-Moon*. The couple walked in the woods and read aloud to one another by firelight. Franklin was drawn to Eleanor by attributes she did not recognize in herself—a willowy, well-proportioned figure, blue eyes, blonde hair, and, most importantly, her sharp intellect and social conscience.

Franklin went to Hyde Park to have his tonsils removed before returning to Harvard that fall. Eleanor was introduced to social activism while working for the National Consumers League, investigating sweatshops where children as young as four were making artificial flowers. She also volunteered at the Rivington Street Settlement House on New York's Lower East Side, teaching dance and calisthenics. She brought Franklin to the slums for a visit to see a sick child and he was taken aback by the abysmal living and working conditions.[32]

In November 1903, Eleanor went to the Harvard-Yale football game in Cambridge. Franklin was a cheerleader. That afternoon, he proposed. Eleanor deferred any immediate commitment to consult with Grandmother Hall, who asked if she was really in love. She found the answer in Elizabeth Barrett Browning's poem, "A Woman's Shortcomings," and incorporated lines from it in a letter to Franklin:

> "Unless you can swear, 'For life, for death!'-
>
> Oh, fear to call it loving!"

Franklin's reply, which Eleanor burned with the rest of his early letters, must have convinced her, though she later confessed to her naivete in young

---

31 Before Theodore Roosevelt took office, the presidential residence was commonly referred to as the Executive Mansion. TR officially named the building "The White House" in 1901 by having the words "The White House – Washington" engraved on his stationary.

32 Miller, 47.

adulthood. "It was years before I understood what being in love was or what loving really means," she wrote.[33]

Franklin now had to break the news to his mother, a task all the more difficult since he had succeeded in concealing the seriousness of the relationship. "I know what pain I must have caused you and you know I wouldn't do it if I could really have helped it," Franklin wrote from Harvard. "Dear Mummy, you know that nothing can ever change what we have always been & always will be to each other—only now you have two children to love and to love you."[34]

Eleanor sent her own self-effacing letter. "I know just how you feel & how hard it must be, but I do so want you to learn to love me a little," she wrote. "You must know that I will always try to do what you wish, for I have grown to love you very dearly during the past summer ... I can only say that my one great wish is always to prove worthy of [Franklin]."[35]

Franklin started Columbia Law School in October 1904 and Sara rented a house on Madison Avenue to share with him. Eleanor received a secret twentieth birthday gift—an engagement ring. "I shall find it hard to keep from wearing it," she wrote her fiancé."[36] Sara had asked the couple to wait a year before announcing the engagement. Franklin planned to break the news to the Delano clan over Thanksgiving dinner at Fairhaven, but fell ill earlier that month, dismissing his symptoms as one of his frequent colds. After a few days, his family physician, Dr. George Draper, diagnosed a liver ailment. The illness, possibly hepatitis A, forced a lengthy absence from Columbia. Eleanor was also sick at the time with "the grippe," a generic term for an upper respiratory tract infection.

When the engagement appeared in newspaper society pages in December 1904, letters of congratulations poured in, including one to the bridegroom from Eleanor's Uncle Theodore. Other family members were more circumspect. Theodore's niece, Corinne Douglas Robinson, felt sorry for her cousin, who had "lived through so much unhappiness, and then to [marry] a man with a mother like Cousin Sally [Sara's family nickname] ... A more determined and possessive woman than I have ever known."[37]

---

33 *Ibid.*, 47.
34 *Ibid.*, 48.
35 Ward, *BTT*, 335.
36 *Ibid.*, 337.
37 *Ibid.*, 337.

Endicott Peabody officiated at the marriage ceremony. Theodore's daughter, Alice, was Eleanor's maid of honor and the President consented to give the bride away, guaranteeing wide press coverage.[38] Rosy was invited to be best man, but was recovering from one of his frequent illnesses, so college roommate Lathrop Brown stepped in.

Attendance at the ceremony on East 76th Street in Manhattan was limited to close friends and relatives. Afterwards, two large doors to the drawing room of the adjoining house were opened and other guests joined the celebration. Theodore marched out to the waiting crowd and almost everyone followed him, leaving the couple of the hour nearly forgotten. "He wants to be the bride at every wedding, the corpse at every funeral, and the baby at every christening," TR's daughter Alice later commented.[39] Despite the pomp, no wedding photograph of the couple has survived.

The newlyweds spent their first week of wedlock at Springwood. For once, Sara left them alone. Their eldest son James later wrote that his father had told him he knew little more than a boy about sex, and Eleanor no more than a little girl. The two had never kissed until after their engagement.

On a three-month honeymoon tour of Europe, Eleanor visited fashionable clothing shops in London and Paris while her husband pursued antiquarian books. Franklin later bragged they stayed in a thousand-dollar-a-night hotel suite, another of his gross exaggerations. He began to call his bride "Babs," short for baby, a term of endearment he used for the rest of their lives. Eleanor became seasick on the voyage home and the ship's doctor explained she was pregnant. "It was quite a relief," she said. "For little fool that I was, I had been seriously troubled for fear that I would never have any children, and my husband would … be much disappointed." Pregnancy gave Eleanor an excuse to avoid marital relations. She later admitted to her daughter she found sex to be "an ordeal to be borne."[40]

38 TR had won election to the presidency in 1904 after assuming it on September 14, 1901, following President McKinley's death from an assassin's bullet.
39 Wead, D., *All the Presidents' Children: Triumph and Tragedy in the Lives of America's First Families.* New York: Atria Books, 2003, 107.
40 Rowley, H., *Franklin and Eleanor: An Extraordinary Marriage.* New York: Picador, 2011, 52.

■ Chapter 3
■ Finding His Way

Franklin returned to Columbia Law School after the honeymoon. The new-lyweds took up residence in a rented Manhattan brownstone on East 36th Street, three blocks from Sara, who announced as a Christmas present that she would be financing construction of a new home for the newlyweds. She had purchased two lots on East 65th Street for twin townhouses. The dwell-ings were to be conjoined, with a shared vestibule and pocket doors connect-ing the upper and lower floor common rooms. Franklin embraced the project, working with architects, builders, and decorators; Eleanor timidly contrib-uted to the plans. After they moved in, Franklin found his bride in tears. The house was not to her liking, she explained. "My husband thought I was quite mad ... and said I would feel different in a little while and left me alone until I should become calmer." she later wrote.[1] "I think he always thought that if you ignored a thing long enough it would settle itself."[2]

Franklin passed the New York State bar exam without having graduated from Columbia and took a job as an unpaid apprentice at Carter, Ledyard, and Milburn, a firm specializing in defending large corporations against antitrust actions. By his second year he was managing clerk, but made no secret that the law was not his life's work, explaining to a group of young lawyers at the firm how he would be following the path his uncle Theodore had taken to the White House. He would first win a seat in the New York State Assembly, then engineer an appointment to be Assistant Secretary of the Navy, and go on to become Governor of New York. "Anyone who is governor of New York has a good chance to be president," Franklin said. Unlike the Sohier family's dismis-sive reaction years earlier, no one "deprecated his ambition or even smiled at it as we might have done," a former colleague observed. "No one had laughed" and FDR's "engaging frankness ... It seemed proper and sincere and moreover, and as he put it, entirely reasonable."[3]

Franklin's forecasted quest for the White House began in 1910, when he was approached by his late father's friend, Dutchess County district attorney John

---

1 Smith, J.E., 55.
2 *Ibid.*
3 Smith, J.E., 59.

E. Mack, about pursuing a safely Democratic Assembly seat. The incumbent, said to be retiring, changed his mind and he was offered the nod for the State Senate instead.

Election to the Senate was anything but a sure thing. A Democrat hadn't held the seat since 1856.[4] The Republican incumbent had prevailed by a two to one margin in the previous election. Poughkeepsie, the district's largest city, was solidly Democratic but the rural areas were hardline Republican.

Franklin rented a bright red Maxwell automobile, a sporty open-air model sure to attract crowds. He peppered his stump speech with good-government generalities and assumed Theodore's pince-nez and mannerisms. Longtime friends were recruited for help. One was Thomas F. Lynch, the son of a Poughkeepsie florist. Lynch set aside two bottles of Champagne and declared he would open them when Franklin was nominated for President. The promise was fulfilled twenty-two years later.

Franklin rode the coattails of a national Democratic landslide to a resounding victory. The state senate met for ten weeks a year. The annual salary was just $1,500 ($47,000 in 2022) and most legislators rented rooms in hotels or boardinghouses while in session. But Franklin had promised his constituents to work for them "twelve months of the year," so the Roosevelt family moved into a stately Albany townhouse built by Martin Van Buren, the first New York governor to be elected President of the United States.[5]

In 1911, United States Senators were still being chosen by state legislatures and New York had designated its combined Assembly and Senate to fill the two seats. One of them, held by Republican Chauncey Depew, was in play. The legislative vote count was about 200, of which 114 were Democrats, so the only uncertainty was which member of their party to choose for the job. Tammany's man was William F. "Blue-Eyed Billy" Sheehan, a one-time lieutenant governor and former political boss of Erie County, now practicing law in New York City. Sheehan's clientele included utility companies that used him as a conduit for contributions to the machine.

To Franklin, Sheehan represented the clubhouse politics and bossism his uncle Theodore disdained, so he decided he owed it to his constituents to oppose him. Twenty like-minded Democrats joined him on the first ballot, preventing

---

4 The 26th District was composed of parts of Dutchess, Putnam, and Columbia counties.
5 *Ibid.*, 70.

either Sheehan or Depew from gaining a majority. Though Franklin hadn't organized the revolt, his name, good looks, and manorial Albany residence made him the face of the insurgency, a role he gleefully embraced. "Tall, with a well set up figure, he is physically fit to command," the New York *Globe* gushed.[6] "With his handsome face and his form of supple strength he could make a fortune on the stage and set the matinee girl's heart throbbing," *The New York Times* wrote.[7]

Unaccustomed to having his will defied, Tammany leader Charles Murphy leaned on the upstarts. All other legislation was set aside. Bankers and wealthy constituents threatened to sanction any legislator who spurned the Tammany candidate. The rebels held firm for sixty-four ballots over ten weeks. In the end, newly elected Governor John Alden Dix, worried that no budget had been passed, called on Sheehan to withdraw. Murphy put up a substitute— State Supreme Court Justice James Aloysius O'Gorman, another former Tammany leader with unimpeachable credentials.

Franklin wanted to hold out for a better choice but a majority of his allies had had enough. The overpowered upstarts arrived for the final vote to jeers and laughter as their opposition broke into the Tammany victory song. But Franklin spun the episode as a triumph, telling an audience, "We have chosen a man for the people who will be dictated to by no one."[8] The "big fight," as he liked to call it, had brought him national renown.[9] Years later he called Sheehan's defeat a victory for good government.

Franklin reprised his gaslighting later in 1911. A blaze at the Triangle Shirtwaist Factory in Manhattan on March 25 had killed 146 workers, mostly young women and children, after the company's owner chained the sweatshop's fire doors shut. In response, two Tammany men, Assembly and Senate leaders Robert F. Wagner and Alfred E. Smith, formed a joint committee to draw up legislation that mandated a maximum fifty-four-hour work week and other measures to improve working conditions.[10] Labor lobbyist Frances Perkins distinctly recalled Franklin's refusal to support the effort. He skipped

6 *Ibid.,* 73.
7 Alter, J., The Defining Moment *FDR's Hundred Days and the Triumph of Hope.* New York: Simon & Schuster, 2007, 33.
8 *Ibid.,* 76.
9 Smith, J.E., 76.
10 Caro, R., *The Power Broker: Robert Moses and the Fall of New York.* New York: Vintage Books, 1975, 128.

the vote and the bill passed solely as a result of Tammany strong-arming.[11] But Franklin again turned the truth upside down, announcing it was he and Wagner who had made the difference. The machine had had enough. In June 1911, after Franklin opposed a highway bill endorsed by leadership, he was voted out of the Democratic caucus.

A few days after the ouster, State Senator Roosevelt collapsed with a 104 degree temperature, swollen throat, and throbbing sinuses from a bacterial infection. No effective treatment existed. When his symptoms began to abate, Eleanor took the children to Campobello, leaving Sara behind as nurse.[12] The condition relapsed and Eleanor returned to Hyde Park to lend support. After another three weeks of recuperation, and a 10-lb weight loss, Franklin returned to the Senate with a plan to cut Tammany's power by advocating for a direct primary to nominate candidates for the U.S. Senate.

In 1912, Franklin joined progressive-minded Democrats in support of New Jersey Governor Woodrow Wilson's candidacy for president. A split in the Republican party augured well for Democrats. Republican incumbent William Howard Taft won renomination from party regulars despite a challenge by Theodore Roosevelt, who had stalked out of the convention and formed his own progressive party. Soon afterwards, TR was delivering a campaign speech in Milwaukee, Wisconsin when a would-be assassin shot him. An iron spectacles case and a folded manuscript in his pocket kept the slug from penetrating deep into TR's chest.

The Democrats convened in Baltimore in late June 1912. The front-runner was the House Speaker, Missourian Champ Clark, though Wilson came with considerable support from primaries. In the Tammany doghouse, Franklin had no official status. Nonetheless, he procured a seat on the convention floor to mix with delegates from across the country. One was a fellow Wilson supporter, North Carolina newspaperman Josephus Daniels. "At that convention Franklin and I became friends—a case of love at first sight," Daniels later wrote.[13]

Nomination required a two-thirds plurality. On the first ballot, Clark failed to gain even a majority. On the ninth ballot, the Tammany machine put its weight behind him but the endorsement backfired. The leader of the

11 Smith, J.E., 81.
12 Ward, G., *A First-Class Temperament.* New York: Harper and Row, 1989, 156.
13 Caro, 93.

party's liberal wing, three-time presidential nominee William Jennings Bryan, stood in opposition, condemning Clark as the candidate of Wall Street. After Bryan threw his support to Wilson and backroom deals were cut over the vice-presidential nominee, Wilson carried the day on the forty-sixth ballot—the most since 1860.

The Roosevelt family now included Anna, born in May 1906, James in December 1907, and Elliott in September 1910. The first Franklin Roosevelt Jr. had been born in March 1909 but died that November of a heart ailment. At Campobello, Franklin was the ringleader of a pint-sized tribe he took sailing, fishing, and climbing seaside cliffs. Franklin preferred the role of playmate to that of disciplinarian. Lacking any good model of motherhood, Eleanor struggled to manage her offspring amid competition from her domineering, intrusive, and often openly critical mother-in-law. "I had never any interest in dolls and little children and I knew absolutely nothing about handling or feeding a baby. What I should have done was to have no servants in those first few years … Had I done this, my subsequent troubles would have been avoided and my children would have had far happier childhoods."[14]

Franklin was champing at the bit to start his Senate reelection campaign that September, but once again illness intervened. On the return trip from Campobello, the shipboard water supply in the Roosevelts' stateroom was contaminated with *Salmonella* bacteria and both Franklin and Eleanor came down with typhoid fever—his case far more severe. The illness brought Franklin a very significant positive consequence—a political genius who would mentor him to the presidency.

Unable to campaign due to profound weakness, Franklin remembered from his earlier days in Albany an odd-looking journalist turned would-be political operative who had asked him for a job. To say the least, Louis McHenry Howe cut a strange figure. A fragile asthmatic as a child, he stood little more than five feet tall. His clothing was rumpled and he reeked from the ashes of Sweet Caporal cigarettes. His face bore the scars of a boyhood bicycle accident. Someone had labeled him a "medieval gnome" and he reveled in that description. Howe's bare-knuckled cynicism about politics masked a deep ambition to hitch his wagon to a great man. After observing Franklin in the state senate, Howe decided he had found him. A hallmark of Franklin's career was his ability to hire the right person for a job. He never made a better choice than Howe.

---

14 Roosevelt, E., *This Is My Story.* New York: Harper & Brothers, 1937, 142–146.

With Franklin flat on his back, Howe orchestrated a campaign on behalf of an invisible candidate. He rented the same car Franklin had used in 1910 and distributed stamped self-addressed questionnaires around the district in order to poll constituents about what concerned them. Using the results, Howe drafted letters over Franklin's signature—promising fishermen lower license fees, apple growers a standardized barrel smaller than currently mandated, and farmers protection from commission merchants who charged them for guiding their crops to urban markets. He also took out newspaper ads that pledged Franklin to a variety of progressive causes, some new for him—women's suffrage and organized labor. Franklin's absence from the campaign trail was never an issue.

Due to split opposition, Franklin won the election by an even larger margin than two years earlier.[15] "Congratulations on your deserved and notable victory," Franklin's Dutchess county friend John Walker wrote. "When a bull moose and an elephant are both outrun by a man sick-a-bed it would seem 'Manifest Destiny.'"[16] Howe addressed his letter of congratulations to the "Beloved and Revered Future President."[17]

A noticeably frail Franklin returned to Albany in January 1913 and was named chairman of the Senate Agriculture Committee. "I'm very well and taking care of myself," he wrote Eleanor. "Wearing rubbers, brushing my teeth, etc., etc." On February 15, an agriculture and farm efficiency expert wrote State Senator Roosevelt to ask him to provide a letter of introduction to his Hudson Valley neighbor, Vincent Astor. Franklin complied, while also expressing a desire to meet with Astor "in regard to improving agricultural methods through co-operation among the farmers of Dutchess County."[18] Farming was only one of the interests the men shared. Roosevelts and the Astors had been intertwined since Franklin's half-brother Rosy married Vincent's Aunt Helen in 1880. Franklin was eight years older than Vincent but by 1913 they had "grown to be the same age."[19] It was the beginning of a highly consequential lifelong friendship.

---

15 The amount of votes garnered by Franklin was virtually the same as 1910 but the Progressive Party candidate's 2600 votes increased the margin of victory. Smith, J.E., 140.
16 Walker to FDR, November 7, 1912.
17 Stiles, L., *The Man Behind Roosevelt*. New York. World Publishing Company, 1954, 25.
18 FDR to Vincent Astor, February 18, 1910. The letter refers to John Davison as the man who is being introduced. Interestingly, the "D." in John D. Rockefeller stands for Davison. FDR Library.
19 Vincent Astor to Missy LeHand June 23, 1937. Missy LeHand files, FDR Library.

Vincent was the son of John Jacob Astor IV, one of the principal heirs to the vast fortune of his namesake great-grandfather. The patriarch Astor had worked his way up as a fur trader and real-estate investor to become the wealthiest man in America. On April 5, 1912, Astor IV went down on RMS *Titanic* and left the bulk of his estate to Vincent, then a twenty-year-old Harvard freshman.

Four years earlier, Astor IV had designated his brother-in-law and close friend, Rosy Roosevelt, as executor of his estate. Assuming that role after Astor's death, Rosy assigned Franklin and his law partner, Langdon P. Marvin, to represent Astor family members in the probate litigation, which included Vincent, still a minor under the law.

Wilson had also won the presidency by virtue of a split of the Republican vote between TR and Taft. Franklin now had a golden opportunity for a spot in the new administration. He wound up serving only two months of his second term in the state senate. After declining offers for Deputy Secretary of the Treasury and Collector of the Port of New York, on March 4, 1913, he ran into Wilson's new Secretary of the Navy, newspaperman Josephus Daniels, at Washington's Willard Hotel during the inauguration celebration. Unfamiliar with maritime affairs, Daniels offered Franklin the job of Assistant Secretary on the spot—"It is singular that I never thought of any other man in that connection," he noted in his diary on March 15.[20] Daniels's newspaper, the Raleigh, North Carolina, *News & Observer*, headlined Franklin's posting "He's Following in Teddy's Footsteps." Daniels ran the appointment past Republican New York Senator and former Secretary of State Elihu Root, who warned him, "Whenever a Roosevelt rides, he wishes to ride in front."[21]

The Navy Department shared a Second Empire wedding cake edifice west of the White House, now known as the Executive Office Building, with the Departments of State and War. Soon after starting work there, Franklin posed with his new boss as the two men stood on an upper porch facing east. Daniels showed the photo to his Assistant Secretary and inquired why the younger man was smiling more broadly than he. Franklin was slow to answer. "I will tell you," Daniels interjected. "We are looking down on the White House and you are saying to yourself, being a New Yorker, 'Someday I will be living in that

---

20 Diary of Josephus Daniels, *Wilson Era*, 124.
21 Smith, J.E., 143.

house'—while I, being from the South, know I must be satisfied with no such ambition."[22,23]

22 Brands, 75.
23 North Carolinian Daniels was an avowed racist. It would not be the last time Franklin was forced to accommodate the social policies of "Dixiecrats" to advance his own agenda.

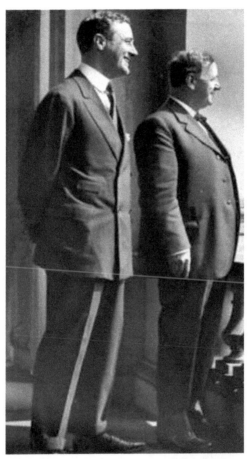

Secretary of the Navy Josephus Daniels and Assistant Secretary Franklin D Roosevelt overlooking the White House from the executive office building, ca. 1914

■ Chapter 4
■ Going to Washington

Despite his sub-cabinet-level position, Franklin became well known around the capital. His keen memory for facts and figures impressed Congressional committees. Navy brass loved him because of his deep knowledge of that service and his hawkish stance about preparedness for war. On the other hand, his cracks about Daniels irked others in the administration. After mocking his boss as "the funniest-looking hillbilly I had ever seen," Franklin drew a rebuke from Interior Secretary Franklin Lane. "Mr. Daniels is your superior," Lane admonished him. "You should show him loyalty or you should resign your office."[1]

Franklin brought Louis Howe with him to Washington as his informal press agent and publicist. At the end of 1913, the Roosevelt family moved into a house at 1733 N Street NW that belonged to Eleanor's Aunt Bamie. "Auntie Bye" was considered to be among the shrewdest of the Oyster Bay Roosevelts. Her brother Theodore rarely made important decisions without her input and her residence became known around Washington as "The Little White House."

A novice to Washington society, Eleanor was in need of a social secretary. At Bamie's recommendation, she hired Lucy Mercer, the twenty-three-year-old daughter of a prominent Maryland family whose patriarch had fallen on hard times. Lucy was beautiful, relaxed, graceful, and sophisticated. "She was femininely gentle where Mother had something of a schoolmarm's charm about her, outgoing where Mother was an introvert," the Roosevelts' son Elliott recalled. "We children welcomed the days she came to work."[2]

In 1913, Franklin was taught an important political lesson. On April 8, Congress had ratified the seventeenth amendment to the Constitution, which mandated direct primary elections for the U.S. Senate. Franklin declared his candidacy for a New York seat. Out of friendship, Daniels agreed to keep Franklin's job open at the Navy Department while he was campaigning. Tammany Boss Murphy backed another member of the Wilson administration—ambassador

---

1 Alter, 42.
2 Roosevelt, E., *An Untold Story*. New York: G.P Putnam's Sons, 1973, 73.

to Germany James W. Gerard, who walloped Franklin in the primary by nearly a three-to-one margin. Franklin spun the crushing defeat by claiming to have carried a majority of New York's counties, declaring he had lost due to Tammany's iron grip on New York City. In truth he had carried just 22 of 61.[3] The upstart learned that any advance in New York politics depended on Tammany's support. Never again did he openly oppose the machine,[4] though he later took measures to punish Gerard for opposing him.[5]

President Wilson's wife, the former Ellen Axson, died on July 28, 1914, a little over a week after the outset of World War I. She had been afflicted with chronic kidney failure and severely elevated blood pressure, then known as Bright's disease. Her passing shattered the president just as he was trying to steer the United States around a European war pitting Germany, Turkey, and the Austro-Hungarian Empire against Russia, France, Britain, and Italy. Wilson adopted a stance of American neutrality.

After the conflict devolved into a bloody trench-bound stalemate across France, Belgium, and Germany, action shifted to the seas, which were dominated by the British navy. Germany turned to submarine warfare as an equalizer. The *Unterseeboot*, or "U-boat," became the scourge of British warships and supply vessels.

On May 7, 1915, a U-boat sank the passenger liner RMS *Lusitania* off the Irish coast, killing 128 Americans. In consequence, the Germans promised to restrict submarine warfare. Wilson upgraded the neutrality policy to one of preparedness. Still, his restraint drew vehement criticism from Republicans including former President Theodore Roosevelt. Franklin publicly supported Wilson.

On July 1, 1915, Franklin underwent emergency surgery for acute appendicitis, a not infrequently fatal affliction in the pre-antibiotic era. He was discharged from the hospital on July 18, then transported aboard his naval yacht to Campobello for five weeks of convalescence.[6] Once back at work, he focused

---

3 Smith, J.E., 124.
4 In 1915, FDR supported the Tammany candidate for sheriff of New York County, Alfred E. Smith.
5 A loyal Democrat, Gerard was denied numerous well-deserved diplomatic appointments during FDR's presidential administrations.
6 Lomazow, S., Fettmann, E., *FDR's Deadly Secret*. New York: Public Affairs: 2010, 19–20.

on preparations for war by creating a Naval Reserve to match a similar force that had been established by the army.

Wilson had come to rely on his presidential physician as a sounding board and personal adviser. Navy doctor Cary Travers Grayson, seasoned by years of service at the White House, made every effort to comfort his patient and commander in chief. Grayson's fiancée, Alice Gertrude Gordon, had befriended a widowed capital socialite she thought might make a good match for the bereft leader. Forty-two-year-old Edith Bolling Galt had been running an exclusive downtown Washington jewelry store bequeathed to her by her late husband. In March 1915, Grayson and Wilson's cousin, Helen Bones, facilitated introductions. Romance blossomed.[7] Grayson was best man when Wilson and Galt wed on December 8, 1915. *The New York Times* reported the presidential physician was Wilson's "closest confidante and friend."

The Kaiser fully unleashed his submarine force on January 7, 1917, hoping to do so with time for the Central Powers to prevail before the United States could mount a meaningful response—but multiple attacks on American vessels caused President Wilson to sever diplomatic relations, then ask for a formal declaration of war on April 6. TR encouraged Franklin to resign and enlist but Wilson vetoed the idea. "Tell the young man to stay where he is," he told Navy Secretary Daniels.[8]

Franklin devised a plan to neutralize the U-boat menace by mining the sea lanes that connected German ports and the North Sea—though he was well aware that the use of mines was a violation of an act ratified at the Hague Convention of 1907 to which the United States was a signatory. Moreover, before America entered the war, Wilson's government had urged Britain and Germany to refrain from such tactics.[9] Nonetheless, Franklin ordered 100,000

---

7 Wilson and Grayson "ran into" Edith coming off a White House elevator after returning from a golf game. "I turned a corner and met my fate" is how Edith later described the meeting in her memoir. She had been attending a tea with Wilson's cousin, Helen Bones, who promptly invited the men to join them. Historians have speculated the meeting was orchestrated by Bones and Grayson to lift the morale of the depressed widower. Edith was the best friend of Grayson's fiancée (Deppisch, L.W., *The White House Physician: A History from Washington to George W. Bush*. Jefferson, NC: McFarland & Company: 2007, 92.) Wilson and Edith spent the remainder of the afternoon chatting and it was not long before invitations came to her for dinners, and car rides. https://www.longwharf.org/woodrow-edith-and-the-lusitania.

8 Davis, 460.

9 Smith, J.E., 143–444.

of the submersible weapons built. Some 70,000 had been deployed by the armistice in November 1918 with at best minimal effect on the war's outcome. Still, Franklin rationalized, "It would not be too far-fetched to say that the North Sea mine barrage had something definite to do with the German naval mutiny, the subsequent army mutiny, and the ending of the war."[10]

Franklin took advantage of the political patronage his position gave him, frequenting naval bases and propitiating key members of Congress. One was Tammany stalwart and House Appropriations Committee chairman John J. Fitzgerald, whose district included the Brooklyn Navy Yard. Cozying up to one-time foes resulted in an invitation to deliver the keynote speech at Tammany's 1917 Independence Day celebration. "I guess we can stand having you, if you can stand coming," said Tammany sachem Daniel J. Riordan, who had delivered the request.[11,12]

Franklin's home life was not going so smoothly. After the birth of the couple's sixth child, John, in March 1916, Eleanor had had enough of pregnancy and therefore of sex. Before long, her handsome, virile thirty-four-year-old husband was paying closer attention to Lucy Mercer. A cat-and-mouse game between the Roosevelts ensued and the Franklin/Lucy relationship became a hot topic for Washington gossip mongers. Alice Roosevelt Longworth spotted the couple in a car in rural Virginia and confronted her cousin. "I saw you twenty miles out in the country but you didn't see me," she said. "Your hands were on the wheel, but your eyes were on that perfectly lovely lady." According to Alice, Franklin responded, "Isn't she perfectly lovely?"[13]

In June 1917, Franklin took Eleanor and a party of friends for a cruise on the Potomac aboard the presidential yacht *Sylph*. The guest list included Lucy, who was ostensibly accompanied by Nigel Law, a handsome near-contemporary of hers from the British embassy. A week later Eleanor fired Lucy, using the excuse that with a war on she had no need of a social secretary.[14] "But if she hoped that by gently letting go her social secretary she would keep Franklin and Lucy from each other, she was to be disappointed," Geoffrey C. Ward wrote. "For on June 24, barely a week after her trip on the Potomac with

---

10 Black, C., *Franklin Delano Roosevelt, Champion of Freedom*. New York: Public Affairs, 2003, 88.
11 Smith, J.E., 145.
12 *Ibid.*
13 Persico, J., *Franklin and Lucy*. New York: Random House, 2008, 107.
14 *Ibid.*, 96.

the Roosevelts, Lucy enlisted in the Navy as a Yeomanette, third class and was assigned to Franklin's secretarial pool at the Navy Department."[15]

A suspicious Eleanor delayed her departure for Campobello until mid-July. Pleading a heavy workload, Franklin was on the island that summer for just ten days. One of his letters to Eleanor from Washington makes mention of another *Sylph* excursion with Lucy Mercer, her beard Nigel Law, and presidential physician Cary Travers Grayson accompanied by his fiancée. Law was later quoted that he took it as a compliment to their friendship that Franklin, "a man I loved and admired," had confided his feelings for Lucy to him.[16]

By this time, Franklin and Lucy were involved in an indiscreet, full-fledged affair. Former vice president Levi Morton's daughter, Edith Morton Eustis, once a Hyde Park neighbor, provided Corcoran House, her stately Washington mansion, as a trysting place. Alice Roosevelt did likewise.[17] "Franklin deserved a good time, he was married to Eleanor," Alice said many decades later.[18]

In August, Eleanor received word that Franklin had taken ill. Leaving the children with Sara, she rushed to a Washington hospital to find her husband with a raging fever from a peritonsillar abscess, a serious throat infection that posed a risk of asphyxiation from a blocked airway. Eleanor returned to Campobello with a promise from Franklin to rejoin the family as soon as he had recovered. "I hated to leave you yesterday," she wrote to him en route. "Please go to the doctor twice a week, eat well and sleep well and remember I count on seeing you on the 26th. My threat was no idle one." Son Elliott later wrote: "There was no mystery; she threatened to leave him."[19] Within a week, Franklin was off on another romantic weekend in Virginia with Lucy and the Graysons.[20]

Lucy was discharged from the Navy on October 5, 1917, "by special order of the Secretary of the Navy"—most likely after the puritanical Daniels got wind of the affair. Whether or not Eleanor tipped him off is unknown. The affair continued.

15 Ward, *FCT*, 367.
16 Persico, 97.
17 Ward, *FCT*, 366.
18 *New York Times Magazine*, August 6, 1967.
19 Smith, J.E., 156.
20 *Ibid.*

Franklin spent the ensuing months gallivanting around Washington with Lucy and Livingston "Livy" Davis, his "good-time Charlie" friend from Harvard whom he had given a job at the Navy Department[21]—all the while lobbying Daniels and Wilson to send him "over there" for a taste of the war in Europe. He got his chance in the summer of 1918, crossing the Atlantic aboard a newly commissioned destroyer, USS *Dyer*. As Daniels's representative, Franklin met with King George and high-ranking British officials. He toured the battlefield at Belleau Wood, where 1800 American marines and infantrymen gave their lives to halt German advances. "We had to thread our way up the steep slope over outcropping rocks, overturned boulders, downed trees, hastily improvised shelter pits, rusty bayonets, broken guns, emergency ration tins, hand grenades, discarded overcoats, rain-stained love letters, crawling lines of ants and many little mounds, some wholly unmarked, some with a rifle bayonet stuck down in the earth, some with a helmet, and some, too, with a whittled cross with a tag of wood or wrapping paper hung over it and, in a pencil scrawl, an American name," he wrote in his diary.[22] The highlight of Franklin's time in France was a meeting with Prime Minister Georges Clemenceau. He also made a point of taking Livy Davis to party with him and his friend Vincent Astor, then occupying the influential position of Port Officer of Royon.[23]

In 1918, a pandemic of "Spanish" influenza spread worldwide.[24] The virus, today known as H1N1, selectively struck young adults. Franklin was not spared. Even before boarding troop transport *Leviathan* for his trip home, he came down with a fever, then collapsed on the ship with double pneumonia and spent the voyage shivering and delirious in his bunk. Shipmates who died of the illness were buried at sea.

Alerted Franklin was sick, Sara, Eleanor, and a doctor were waiting when *Leviathan* reached New York. Franklin was carried off the ship on a stretcher to an ambulance for transport to the family townhouses on East 65th Street. While unpacking his suitcase, Eleanor found a sheaf of letters from Lucy Mercer to her husband. "The bottom dropped out of my own particular

---

21 Franklin appointed Davis head of "Eyes for the Navy" a program he devised whereupon private citizens were paid a dollar to loan binoculars for military use. As silly as this may sound, the program had a modicum of success. The binoculars were returned to their owners after the war.

22 Friedel, F., *Franklin D. Roosevelt, A Rendezvous With Destiny*. New York and Boston: Back Bay Books, 1990, 30–31.

23 Diary of FDR, August 15, 1918, FDRL.

24 The virus did not originate in Spain, but got its name because the country was one of few that enjoyed a free press and was able to openly report it.

world," she told an interviewer after Franklin's death. "I faced myself, my surroundings, my world, honestly for the first time."[25]

Most sources suggest Eleanor offered Franklin a divorce, but he came to his senses after Sara threatened to cut off his finances and Louis Howe told him the scandal would end his political career.[26,27] Divorce or overt marital discord were nonstarters.

No Roosevelt had ever been divorced.[28] In 1912, Alice had expressed a desire to leave her philandering alcoholic husband, Nicholas Longworth. "I don't think one can have any idea how horrendous even the idea of divorce was in those days," she later wrote. The usually irrepressible Alice stayed married.[29]

James later gave his version of the agreement his parents reached in 1918. They would "go on for the sake of appearances, the children, and the future, but as business partners, not as husband and wife, provided he end his affair with Lucy at once, which he agreed to do … after that, Father and Mother had an armed truce that endured to the day he died."[30] Anything James or his brother Elliott wrote about their parents has to be taken with a grain of salt, but clearly an arrangement was reached which would facilitate Franklin's political career. The Mercer affair brought about the Roosevelts' first and most enduring deception—the charade of a traditional marriage.

---

25 Miller, 152.
26 Persico, 124, 128.
27 Some historians have speculated that Lucy's Catholic faith, which barred divorce, was a factor, but, as Joseph Persico's authoritative account notes, Lucy's father was an Episcopalian and her Catholic mother had been divorced before she married him. A credible, recently discovered second-hand account may provide an additional scenario: Eleanor "flatly refused to give [Franklin] a divorce under any circumstances then or in the future and that was that. Evidently because of his political ambitions Franklin Roosevelt was forced to abide by this edict and of course at the time fear of scandal was an important consideration." Guy Castle related the story told him by his mother and also includes a verifiable anecdote about how Lucy's sister, Violetta, committed suicide after discovering the infidelity of her physician husband. Letter of Guy Castle. Westbrook Pegler Papers. Herbert Hoover Library.
28 The stigma of divorce apparently ended with FDR's five children, who had nineteen marriages and fifteen divorces between them.
29 Alice took the matter into her own hands, taking up with another serial philanderer, Senator William Borah, known around Washington as the "Idaho Stallion." It became common knowledge that her child was fathered by Borah and Alice was saddled with the sobriquet "Aurora Borah Alice." Persico, 109.
30 Asbell, B., ed., *Mother and Daughter*. New York: Fromm International Publishing, 1988, 26.

Once recovered from the flu, Franklin again petitioned Wilson to let him enlist but the President told him there was no need as the war would soon be over. Hostilities ended on November 11, 1918.

Wilson went to Paris for peace talks following the armistice. His entourage included Eleanor and Franklin, who was assigned to negotiate the sale or dismantling of American wartime naval installations. Huge throngs greeted the American President as a visionary who had excited hopes for lasting peace with his "Fourteen Points" plan. One of Wilson's key proposals was for a "League of Nations" to peaceably settle international disputes. He succeeded in getting his brainchild included in the Versailles Treaty, which was signed on June 28, 1919—but the treaty required ratification by the Senate, now controlled by Republicans who viewed participation in the League as a threat to American sovereignty.

Wilson took his case to the people on a grueling nationwide whistle-stop tour. His health had been tenuous since his days as a professor at Princeton and the strain of his latest political battle broke him. He collapsed in Pueblo, Colorado, on September 25, 1919. Taken back to Washington, he suffered a major stroke on October 2. A blocked artery in his brain left him paralyzed on his left side, without left-sided vision and cognitively impaired. At first Dr. Grayson attempted to blame Wilson's collapse in Colorado on Spanish flu. Even after the devastating stroke, he told Secretary of State Robert Lansing that Wilson's mind was "not only clear but active" and his problems were "a touch of indigestion and a depleted nervous system."[31] Barred from seeing Wilson, Vice President Thomas Marshall hesitated to move into the role for which his position existed.

With Grayson's collaboration, Edith Wilson began an elaborate cover-up. The First Lady composed her husband's letters and orders and guided his hand as he "signed" them. A meeting was staged to obviate growing concern among members of the cabinet and Congress. Wilson's paralyzed left side was

---

31 Lomazow, S. and Fettmann. E. *FDR's Deadly Secret*, New York: Public Affairs, 2010, 21.

obscured and the officials were seated to his right.[32] The ploy was successful. The cover-up lasted for the remaining eighteen months of Wilson's term.[33]

Franklin's principal concern at the 1920 Democratic convention in San Francisco was, as always, his own political future. With passage of the nineteenth amendment to the Constitution anticipated, women would be voting for the first time and he surmised that his looks and charm might be helpful in a campaign. Tammany Boss Murphy put forth Al Smith as a favorite son candidate for president. Franklin seconded the nomination. Frances Perkins recalled the way he "displayed his athletic ability by vaulting over a row of chairs to get to the speaker's podium."[34,35]

The strongest Democratic candidate was Wilson's son-in-law, William Gibbs McAdoo, but the stroke-addled president purposely deadlocked the convention in the hope his party would call on him to run for a third term. A compromise candidate, Governor James Cox of Ohio, was nominated on the forty-fourth ballot. The next day, Cox told his campaign manager he wanted Franklin as his running mate, reasoning that New York State had the most electoral college votes, and the Roosevelt name might be an asset. The selection required Tammany's endorsement. Boss Murphy held his nose and acceded. "This young Roosevelt is no good, but if you want him go ahead and we'll vote for him," Murphy declared.[36,37]

Franklin was now on a national ticket at age 38, four years younger than TR had been when he ran for vice president. Well aware that Democratic chances in 1920 were a long shot at best, he used his candidacy to introduce himself to Americans across the country by giving more than a thousand speeches, sometimes being called out by Republicans for his exaggerations.[38] He also built a political cadre. One of the first to sign on, as advance man, was Stephen T. Early,

---

32 Wilson sustained an occlusion of the major artery supplying blood to his nondominant right cerebral hemisphere, which left him with dense paralysis of his left arm and leg and loss of left sided vision. As often happens with severe nondominant hemispheric stroke syndromes, he also had anosognosia, the inability to recognize he had suffered a stroke at all. This is evidenced by the fact that, even in his severely disabled state, he expressed a desire to run for a third term.
33 Even after his term ended, Grayson *never* publicly admitted Wilson had suffered a stroke.
34 Smith, J.E., 179.
35 Perkins, F., *The Roosevelt I Knew*. New York: Viking Press, 1946, 27.
36 Smith, J.E., 180.
37 Black, 124.
38 One of the most flagrant was that he had written the constitution of Haiti.

who had become acquainted with Franklin and Louis Howe while in Albany as an Associated Press reporter. Another newshound, Marvin H. McIntyre, became the campaign's publicity chief and business manager. Formerly editor of the *Washington Times*, McIntyre resigned from that position in 1917 to become a special assistant to Josephus Daniels at the Department of the Navy. Another pillar of the Roosevelt campaign organization was Marguerite Alice LeHand, a bright, ambitious Irish Catholic from the blue-collar Boston suburb of Somerville, Massachusetts. LeHand, later known as "Missy,"[39] was hired at the recommendation of Franklin's campaign chairman, Charles H. McCarthy,[40] who had grown to appreciate her outstanding professional and social skills after he hired her for a job at the Navy Department.[41]

Early in their campaign, Franklin and Cox paid Wilson a visit to assure him of their support for the League of Nations. "As we came in sight of the [White House] we saw the President in a wheel chair, his left shoulder covered with a shawl which concealed his left arm, which was paralyzed," Franklin wrote decades later. "His utter weakness was startling and I noticed tears in the eyes of Cox."[42]

Cox pushed ratification of the Versailles Treaty and its League of Nations at a nation fatigued with talk of international relations. The Republican candidate, Ohioan Warren G. Harding, a randy former newspaper publisher turned United States senator, embraced the slogan "A Return to Normalcy."

Normalcy won by a landslide. Harding received a staggering sixty-one percent of the popular vote and carried every state outside the South. Republicans won lopsided victories in the House and Senate. In New York, Democrats took just 27 percent of the vote, losing every statewide office down ballot.

Cox retired from the politics to run a media business, Cox Communications, that grew to become a nationwide conglomerate, but no blot of defeat stained his former running mate. Franklin sought to preserve the core of his staff for the future. At Christmas 1920, he presented key aides with sets of gold cufflinks from Tiffany's, his initials engraved on one, theirs on the other. Henceforth, members of the "Cuff Links Club" comprised the bedrock of

---

39 The moniker came about and stuck after Franklin's youngest child, John, had difficulty calling her "Miss LeHand."
40 McCarthy was an original member of Franklin's cufflinks club.
41 Smith, K., *The Gatekeeper*. New York: Touchstone, 2007, 35.
42 Cox, J., *Journey through My Years*. New York: Simon and Schuster, 1946, 241–242.

his political organization. Missy LeHand, by now indispensable, stayed on as Franklin's personal secretary.

◼ Chapter 5
◼ Disaster

After the election, Franklin took a job as vice president of the Fidelity and Deposit Company, a surety bonding firm run by Democratic kingpin Van Lear Black, owner of *The Baltimore Sun*.[1] He was well suited for the job—soliciting clients from among the well-heeled acquaintances he had made through family, schools, and politics. Louis Howe and Missy LeHand came along with him. Steve Early returned to the Associated Press, then, in 1927, became Washington representative of *Paramount News*, the newsreel division of *Paramount Pictures*. Marvin McIntyre took a position at *Pathé News Reels*.

Franklin emerged from the 1920 election as a proven campaigner with a bright future in the Democratic party, making him a prime political target. In July 1921, a Senate subcommittee made up of two Republicans and one Democrat launched an investigation of one of Franklin's most controversial undertakings while Assistant Secretary of the Navy.

In January 1919, reports of excessive drinking, illicit drug use, and homosexual activity at the Newport, Rhode Island, naval base had come to light. A court of inquiry found the allegations to be justified and the Navy Department began an investigation. Enlisted men were recruited as decoys. Some engaged in sex to entrap other sailors. Arrests began in late April. A three-week trial ended with the court-martial of seventeen sailors for sodomy and "scandalous conduct." Most defendants were sent to naval prison, two were dishonorably discharged. Two were acquitted.[2]

Franklin told the committee that when discovered the "highly improper and revolting methods" of inquiry being used, he ordered them stopped. He also complained about not being given enough time to review the documents to defend himself before the majority report was filed.

---

1 His salary was a whopping $25,000 ($416,000 in 2022). Meier, A. *Morganthau: Power, Privilege, and the Rise of an American Dynasty*. New York: Random House, 2022, 190.
2 https://military-history.fandom.com/wiki/Newport_sex_scandal.

A page 4 headline in *The New York Times* on July 20, 1921, read:

LAY NAVY SCANDAL TO F. D. ROOSEVELT;

Senate Naval Sub-Committee Accuses Him and Daniels in Newport Inquiry

DETAILS ARE UNPRINTABLE

The article presented conflicting arguments about what the Assistant Secretary had known and when he learned it. Franklin defended himself by accusing the committee's majority members of partisanship. "As an American, one deplores bad faith and a conscious perversion of facts on the part of any Senator," he said. "One hates to see the United States Navy used as the vehicle for cheap ward politics ... It rather amuses me that these Republican Senators consider me worthwhile attacking so maliciously and savagely." Had the scandal lingered in the headlines, it might have made political trouble for a rising Democratic star, but medical catastrophe soon rendered that possibility moot.

Two weeks before joining his family at Campobello, Franklin, now 39, had traveled forty miles up the Hudson on the steam yacht *Pocantico* to join 2,100 Boy Scouts camping at Bear Mountain State Park.[3] He emceed a mess-hall chicken dinner, mingled in the crowd, and posed for group snapshots. He returned to New York City for a few days, then headed north with Louis Howe aboard Van Lear Black's yacht, *Sabalo*.

"Infantile paralysis," as polio was commonly known at the time, first became a concern for Franklin in the summer of 1916 when a pandemic of the virus hit New York City with 19,000 cases—2,448 of them fatal. Wealthy parents shipped tens of thousands of their children out of town. Municipalities bordering the city enforced strict quarantines. "NEW YORKERS KEEP OUT. WE SYMPATHIZE BUT WE HAVE CHILDREN," a sign read.

"This awful disease is spreading," Sara wrote her son from Campobello in August 1916. "I trust our little island will be immune." Franklin did not arrive to take his family back to Springwood until the end of September, and then on a three-day voyage aboard his naval yacht *Dolphin*, rather than on the customary crowded public train.[4]

---

3 At the time, Franklin was President of the Greater New York Council of the Boy Scouts of America.
4 Ward, *FCT*, 317–318.

The polio virus infects its victims by being ingested, spreading from feces into the water supply, and, by contact, into food. The incubation period between exposure and onset of symptoms can be up to thirty-five days. Despite numerous accounts of Franklin "catching" polio at Campobello after a swim in the frigid Bay of Fundy,[5] he'd already become infected at Bear Mountain amid the primitive sanitary conditions. By the time he arrived in Canada, his fate had been sealed.[6]

5 The story of Franklin's illness has been told in books, a successful Broadway play and a movie, *Sunrise at Campobello*. The play opened on Broadway in 1958 and ran for 558 performances. (See https://en.wikipedia.org/wiki/ Sunrise at Campobello (play)). FDR was portrayed in a Tony Award-winning performance by Ralph Bellamy, who reprised the role in the Academy Award nominated 1960 film of the same name, directed by Dore Schary. Greer Garson was nominated for an Academy Award for her portrayal of Eleanor. (See https://en.wikipedia.org/wiki/Sunrise_at_Campobello.)
In recent years, two motion pictures have been produced which purport to be based on Franklin's life. The first, *Hyde Park on Hudson* (2012), with Daisy Suckley as the central character, starring Bill Murray as Franklin; the second, *Atlantic Crossing*, produced in 2020 by PBS, centered around his "relationship" with Princess Martha of Norway. Both of these films are so littered with glaring historical gaffe that nothing of any historical value can be gleaned from either of them.

6 Tobin, J., *The Man He Became*. New York: Simon and Schuster, 2013 is a comprehensive and valuable account of Roosevelt's illness. As has been hypothesized by Tobin and again in a recent book by Jonathan Darman, this author does not agree that polio provided Franklin with an infusion of empathy. His deceptive, magnetic personality, incredible intellect, astounding communitive skills and persistence to achieve the presidency were unchanged. He overcame incredible odds to achieve greatness and thrived due to the events that occurred along with his pioneering use of new medium of radio as a political force. Because of his handicap, it took seven long years to get back in the game, and when he did, his health problems were a deterrent rather than an asset.
Tobin describes the importance of spinal fluid analysis to diagnose the disease. Lacking the original laboratory analysis, he ferreted out the evidence to make a convincing argument that the procedure was performed.
The importance of spinal fluid analysis in diagnosing polio cannot be overstated, especially since a group of statistical analysts doggedly continue to cast doubt on Roosevelt's diagnosis, asserting that another condition associated with infection, Guillain-Barre Syndrome (GBS) a condition affecting nerves after an infection, is more likely. FRANKLIN DID NOT HAVE GBS.
In 1916, Georges Guillain, Jean Alexandre Barré, and André Strohl described the diagnostic spinal fluid abnormality of GBS, providing an important means of differentiating GBS from polio. A spinal tap involves the insertion of a long needle between the vertebrae to extract fluid from the sac that surrounds the spinal cord and a portion of the nerves that emanate from it. An elevated white blood cell count in conjunction with a normal protein level in the spinal fluid is a hallmark of the diagnosis of poliomyelitis. As Tobin also explains (p. 67), the notion that a spinal tap was of therapeutic value in treating the disease fell out of favor by the 1930s. Neurologists continue to employ spinal taps as a diagnostic tool for infection and multiple sclerosis. It is used therapeutically to treat a few relatively

Franklin's five children, now six to fifteen,[7] looked forward to the outings their father led them on. After one foray, Franklin returned fatigued. Too tired to change out of his bathing suit or eat, he began feeling chills and went to bed. By morning he was unsteady on his feet, felt "thoroughly achy all over," and had stabbing pains in his legs and a temperature of 102 degrees.[8] A local physician diagnosed a severe cold. The next morning he awoke with rubbery legs. His skin had become sensitive to the point he could not even bear the mild pressure of his bedclothes.[9] As the day progressed, so did the weakness in the muscles of his buttocks, abdomen, and arms. By evening he could not stand or even hold a pencil and was having trouble urinating. Eleanor was co-opted

uncommon disease states to reduce fluid pressure in the brain. The diagnostic hallmark of GBS is "Albumino-cytological dissociation," an increased concentration of spinal fluid protein and a normal (zero) cell count. Patients with acute polio show the opposite profile—an elevated white blood cell count and normal protein levels.

As the scientifically descriptive name acute inflammatory demyelinating polyneuropathy (AIDP) used today implies that the pathology involves the substance that surrounds and enhances the function of peripheral nerves themselves, while the polio virus selectively attacks the anterior horn cells (motor neurons) within the spinal cord, an important distinction. The cardinal consequence of anterior horn cell disease is muscle wasting, which is rarely, if ever, seen in GBS and *never* to the extent manifested in FDR's case. Muscle atrophy due to motor neuron disease is also the hallmark of Amyotrophic Lateral Sclerosis (ALS), commonly known as "Lou Gehrig's Disease."

Franklin's highly competent physicians, Lovett, Levine, and later, George Draper, all had an excellent knowledge of the contemporary medical literature as well as extensive experience with polio, especially after the notorious epidemic that struck New York City in 1916. Present-day neuromuscular disease experts strongly support the diagnosis of polio over GBS due to a number of historical and physical aspects of Roosevelt's illness that included the coincident febrile illness of his children, chills, fever, and achiness contemporaneous with onset of weakness, shooting pain, and early profound lower extremity muscular atrophy with relative sparing of the upper extremities. (Personal communication with John Halperin, M.D., Chairman of Neurosciences, Overlook Hospital, Summit, NJ.) A 2016 paper by three eminent neuromuscular specialists states unequivocally there has *never* been a reported case where a GBS patient became confined to a wheelchair! Ditunno, J.F. Jr., Becker, B.E., Herbison, G.J., "Franklin Delano Roosevelt: The Diagnosis of Poliomyelitis Revisited." *PM&R* 2016;8:883–893.

7 The second Franklin Jr. had been born in August 1914 and John in March 1916.
8 Tobin, J., *The Man He Became.* New York: Simon & Schuster, 2014, 49.
9 Gallagher, H.G., *FDR's Splendid Deception.* New York: Dodd Mead, 1985, 11. Severe skin hypersensitivity has recently been reported with SARS-COVID-19. Krajewswsi, P., Szepietowski, J.C., Maj, J., "Cutaneous Hyperesthesia: A Novel Manifestation of COVID-19." *Brain, Behavior, and Immunity* 2020 July;87:188. It has previously been reported in acute poliomyelitis. "Sensory Losses in Poliomyelitis." Seggey, J., Ohry, A., Rozin, R., Rubinstein, E., "Letter: Sensory Losses in Poliomyelitis." *Archives of Neurology* 1976;33(9):664.

into the role of nurse, bathing and feeding her husband and managing his urinary catheter.

Working the phone, Louis Howe located the venerable Philadelphia neurosurgeon, William Williams Keen, 84, at his summer home in nearby Bar Harbor, Maine.[10] At Campobello, Keen diagnosed "a clot of blood from a sudden congestion" that had "settled in the lower spinal cord, temporarily removing the power to move, though not to feel."[11] He prescribed heavy massage of Franklin's legs and predicted a quick recovery. Keen changed his mind a few days later and wrote Eleanor to offer a different opinion—that Franklin had a far more serious problem—a "lesion of the spinal cord" which carried a far worse long-term prognosis. He also enclosed a bill for $600—$10,000 in 2022.

For ten days, Eleanor and Howe spent hours kneading Franklin's leg muscles. The excruciatingly painful regimen made things worse. Now paralyzed chest to toes, Franklin was slipping in and out of a fevered delirium. Eleanor later wrote that her husband was "out of his head" in a draft of her autobiography. Franklin blue-penciled the phrase from the manuscript.[12]

Louis Howe was first to suspect poliomyelitis and sent a detailed description of Franklin's symptoms to Sara's brother, Frederic Delano, to ask his help in finding a competent physician. The ensuing chain of conversations led to Samuel Levine, an internist at Peter Bent Brigham Hospital in Boston. Hearing Franklin's symptoms, Levine dismissed Keen's diagnosis and said it "seemed clear Mr. Roosevelt was suffering from acute poliomyelitis." Levine recommended a spinal tap [removing fluid in the spinal sac using a long needle between the vertebrae] be performed to confirm the diagnosis and relieve cerebrospinal fluid pressure in hopes of lessening Franklin's paralysis.[13]

---

10 Keen had been one of the surgeons who performed secret surgery to remove a cancerous tumor from President Grover Cleveland's jaw in 1893. He exposed the procedure in an article in The Saturday Evening Post in 1918. For a captivating version of the complete story of the procedure see: Algeo, M., *The President Is a Sick Man: Wherein the Supposedly Virtuous Grover Cleveland Survives a Secret Surgery at Sea and Vilifies the Courageous Newspaperman Who Dared Expose the Truth.* Chicago: Chicago Review Press, 2012.

11 Lomazow and Fettmann, 26.

12 *Ibid.,* 27

13 Levine, S.A., "Some Notes Concerning the Early Days of Franklin D. Roosevelt's Attack of Poliomyelitis and Experience with Other Presidents' Illnesses," unpublished manuscript, quoted in Goldberg, R.T., *The Making of Franklin D. Roosevelt.* Lanham, MD: Natl Book Network, 1991, 30.

When Eleanor confronted Keen with Levine's conclusions, the older doctor reached out for Boston orthopedist Dr. Robert W. Lovett, America's leading authority on infantile paralysis. Lovett came to Campobello, where he confirmed Levine's diagnosis and offered Eleanor a glimmer of hope. "The case was not of the severest type," Lovett said, "and some of the important muscles might be on the edge where they could be influenced towards recovery or become completely paralyzed."[14],[15]

"I'm not going to mention the word 'paralysis' unless I have to," Louis Howe told Eleanor. "If it's printed, we're sunk. His career is *kaput*, it's finished."[16] Thus began a twenty-four-year cover-up of the degree of Franklin's paralysis and disability. Howe slipped some details to the Augusta, Maine, *Daily Kennebec Journal.* That newspaper's August 27, 1921, headline announced, "Franklin Roosevelt Improving After Threat of Pneumonia." He "had been seriously ill at his summer home at Campobello, but is now improving," the article stated. He "took a heavy cold and was threatened with pneumonia but was slightly improved and progressing favorably." This became the mantra for describing Franklin's condition—temporary and improving.

The next task was to get Franklin back to New York City. Sara reached out for her cousin, railroad executive Lyman Delano, who had a private railcar rolled to a siding in nearby Eastport, Maine. The first leg of the trip was by far the most challenging. A team of attendants cocooned him into a stretcher in his second-floor bedroom, then carried him outside and down a steep hill to the wharf. A small boat ferried him across two miles of open water to a sardine dock in Eastport. He was hauled over cobbles on an iron-wheeled baggage cart to the siding where the train was waiting, then loaded aboard his private car through an open window. Louis Howe had diverted reporters assigned to cover the event to the other side of town. By the time they caught up with him, Franklin was in a seat, propped up on pillows—chatting, smiling, and smoking a cigarette in a holder held at a jaunty angle.[17] The six-hundred-mile journey to Manhattan's Grand Central Terminal ended at 3:20 the next afternoon, September 14, 1921. An ambulance transported him twenty-eight blocks uptown to Presbyterian Hospital, only a few blocks from his home on East 65th Street.

---

14 Robert Lovett papers, Harvard, quoted in Smith, J.E., 191–192.
15 Tobin, 2013, 66.
16 Houck, D.W., *Rhetoric as Currency.* College Station: Texas A&M University Press, 2001, 99.
17 Gallagher, 18; Roosevelt, E. and Brough, J, *An Untold Story: The Roosevelts of Hyde Park.* New York: Putnam, 152–153; Ward, *FCT,* 598–599.

■ Chapter 6
■ Fighting Back

On September 15, 1921, the *New York Times* broke the news that Franklin had polio. The article included a knowingly misleading statement by Dr. George Draper, who had assumed responsibility for Franklin's daily care. "You can say definitely that he will not be crippled,"[1] Draper declared, "No one need have any fear of permanent injury from his attack." The newspaper accepted his opinion, writing that while Franklin's illness had affected his legs, "it was said that Mr. Roosevelt would not be permanently crippled" and "for more than a week he has been recovering the use of the affected members."[2]

Too weak to hold a pen, Franklin dictated a letter to *Times* publisher Adolph S. Ochs, in the jovial tone he employed to make light of serious medical problems. "While the doctors were unanimous in telling me that the attack was very mild and that I was not going to suffer any permanent effects from it, I had, of course, the usual dark suspicion that they were just saying nice things to make me feel good," he wrote. "But now that I have seen the same statement officially made in *The New York Times* I feel immensely relieved because I know of course it must be so."[3]

Dr. Draper feared that Franklin might not even recover the ability to hold himself in a sitting position and asked Dr. Lovett to fashion a brace to soften the psychological blow should his patient fail to attain that critical milestone. But after five weeks, Franklin's back muscles were strong enough to support him, the febrile, infectious phase of the disease had ended, and it was deemed safe for him to rehabilitate at home. The move from the hospital took place at night to minimize the chance of anyone seeing him being carried up his front steps on a stretcher. Franklin's bed was outfitted with a trapeze so he could exercise his upper body. His pain eased and his arm strength grew, but his leg muscles remained flaccid.

During the winter of 1921–1922, the twin townhouses at 47–49 East 65th Street were crammed with five children, two nurses often at odds with each

---

1 Tobin, 99.
2 *New York Times*, September 16, 1921.
3 FDR to Ochs, A.S., *FDR Library*. quoted in Smith, J.E., 192–193.

other, and the chain-smoking Louis Howe. For Franklin, the environment was physically and psychologically arduous. A battle developed between Sara, who wanted her son to retire to the sedate life of the country squire, and the team of Eleanor and Howe, who were allied in their belief that Franklin should not abandon his political career. But a man who could barely sit up was by no means ready to make any firm decision about his future.

The polio virus selectively attacks nerves in the spinal cord known as motor neurons, which nourish individual muscles, causing them to shrivel. Left unchecked, this phenomenon can freeze a limb in an abnormal position known as a contracture. In Franklin's case, despite the finest physical therapy, contractures were beginning to distort his hips and legs in a way that would prevent him from standing erect and putting his feet flat on the floor, making it impossible for him to use crutches. As a remedy, doctors encased him in a plaster cast from the waist down. At intervals, wedges were driven into the cast to progressively straighten his spine and joints. Franklin weathered this intensely painful process with stoic optimism. After the cast was removed, he was fitted with waist-to-ankle metal braces that locked and unlocked at the knees. The braces incorporated a leather band to support his pelvis. Using the contraption, Dr. Draper, Eleanor, and two nurses were able to hoist Franklin into a standing position for the first time since he was stricken. There was now at least some hope he could start to learn to use crutches.

At Dr. Draper's insistence, Franklin went to Boston to see Dr. Lovett. During that ten-day stay, technicians modified his braces and "taught him some tricks about getting up and down stairs and walking." Lovett sent his patient home with instructions on how to practice with crutches, though he found little reason to believe Franklin's legs would regain their former strength.[4] They never came close. A good way to understand Lovett's prognosis is to imagine trying to regrow the leaves on tree branches whose roots have been cut.

Dr. Draper recommended that his patient relocate from "the intense and devastating influence of the interplay of those high-voltage personalities" in his household.[5] Sara took her two oldest grandchildren off to Europe and Franklin relocated to Springwood for the summer with Eleanor, Howe, and a nurse to concentrate on building his upper body strength and increase his mobility and endurance.

---

4 Tobin, 148.
5 *Ibid.*

Upon returning from Europe, Sara decided her son needed companion-ship to enliven his boring Hyde Park workouts. Two unmarried female rel-atives—Franklin's first cousin, Laura Franklin "Polly" Delano, and a sixth cousin, Margaret Lynch "Daisy" Suckley, lived nearby. Sara invited them to Springwood. Both became Franklin's lifelong intimate friends. "Mrs. James [Sara] would invite me and others to tea," Suckley recalled, "because Franklin was lonely and needed to see people."[6] He detested the term "infantile paraly-sis," telling Daisy, "I'm not going to be conquered by a childish disease."[7]

Franklin's rehabilitation included twice-a-week trips to nearby Rhinebeck, where Vincent Astor's thousand-acre estate, Ferncliff, sported an indoor swimming pool. Swimming not only strengthened Franklin's body, it ele-vated his spirits. "The water put me where I am and the water has to bring me back!"[8] he told Sara's chauffeur, Louis Depew. "The legs work wonderfully in the water," he wrote Dr. Draper, "and I need nothing to keep myself afloat."[9]

Within a few months, he had bulked up. When a visitor accused him of get-ting fat, he retorted, "the upper part of me weighs, of course, more than it did before, but that is because my arm and shoulder muscles have developed tremendously in this effort of getting about with crutches."[10]

By February 1923, Franklin was being bombarded with recommendations for miracle cures. "You doctors have sure got imaginations," he wrote Dr. Draper. "Have any of your people thought of distilling the remains of King Tut Ankh-Amen? The serum might put new life into some of our mutual friends. In the meantime, I am going to Florida to let nature take its course—nothing like Old Mother Nature, anyway."[11]

Franklin rented a sixty-foot houseboat with a four-man crew and began sail-ing around the Florida Keys. After a few days, Eleanor had had enough of mar-itime life and returned home—but being at sea energized her husband. With his African-American valet, Leroy Jones, to help him get around and Missy LeHand as hostess, Franklin began inviting former law partners, Harvard

6 Ward, *FCT*, 629.
7 Tobin, 148.
8 Roosevelt and Shalett, 162. The cold water of the Bay of Fundy that FDR fell into the day before he became symptomatic with polio did not cause the disease, but FDR liked to tell it that way.
9 Ward, *FCT*, 145.
10 Roosevelt and Shalett, 167.
11 Ward, *FCT*, 680.

schoolmates, and other friends and their wives to join him for irreverent adventures of fishing, sailing, and drinking rum. Even the dour Louis Howe spent a few days on board.[12] Franklin reveled in the experience. He continued to pursue sea-going escapes for the remainder of his life.

Franklin returned to see Dr. Lovett in the spring of 1924. While he had made transitory gains, his legs were weaker than they had been the year before. But his time in Florida had brought a revelation. "I have found ... for myself one interesting fact which I believe to be a real discovery," he wrote to a twenty-seven-year-old polio patient whose recovery had plateaued. "My muscles have improved with greater rapidity when I could give them sunlight. Last winter I went to Florida and was much in the open air under the direct rays of the sun with very few clothes on, and there is no doubt that the leg muscles responded more quickly ... This summer also I have made a real effort to sit in the sun for several hours a day and the improvement has undoubtedly been more rapid," Franklin wrote. "I am confident that with a continuation of plenty of sunlight and exercise I shall be able to get rid of crutches and braces."[13]

Dr. Lovett died "after a few days illness" on July 2, 1924, while vacationing in England.[14] Lacking a medical guru, Franklin pursued new ideas on his own. Schools of thought regarding polio rehabilitation abounded and Franklin did a deep dive into every method he could find. He settled on an approach devised by Dr. James MacDonald, a neurologist recommended by his uncle Fred Delano. "Of course, I have seen the methods of practically all the other doctors—the Lovett Method, Goldthwaite Method, Hibbs Method, St. Louis Method, Chicago Method, etc., etc.," Franklin wrote to Uncle Fred "They are good in their way, but MacDonald uses what they use and goes one step further. The principle of the others is the exercise of individual muscles, primarily in the line of straight pull. MacDonald's exercises give all of this, but in addition exercises in coordination with each other, i.e., the pull outside the direct plane ... In other words MacDonald seeks functioning as the primary objective and he has certainly succeeded in dozens of cases."[15] On October 11, 1924, Franklin wrote to Dr. William Egleston of Hartsville, South Carolina, "The following treatment is so far the best, judging from my own experience and that of hundreds of other cases which I have studied:

---

12 *Ibid.*, 681.
13 FDR to Harry Wilson Walker, July 29, 1924, FDRL.
14 *New York Times*, July 3, 1924.
15 Ward, FCT, 731.

"Gentle exercises especially for the muscles which seem to be worst affected. [He had learned a bitter lesson that overdoing exercise was harmful.]

"Gentle skin rubbing—not muscle kneading—bearing in mind that good circulation is a prime requisite.

"Swimming in warm water—lots of it.

"Sunlight—all the patient can get, especially direct sunlight on the affected parts. It would be ideal to lie in the sun all day with nothing on. This is difficult to accomplish but the nearest approach to it is a bathing suit."[16]

Franklin had also devised an ingenious method to measure his progress. "I still wear braces, of course, because the quadriceps [the muscles that straighten the knee] are not yet strong enough to bear my weight," he told Dr. Egleston. "One year ago I was able to stand in fresh water without braces when the water was up to my chin. Six months ago I could stand in water up to the top of my shoulders and today can stand in water just level with my armpits. This is a very simple method for me of determining how fast the quadriceps are coming back."[17]

In the fall of 1924, Franklin partnered with John Lawrence, a Harvard classmate who was also "crippled in the legs," to buy their own houseboat. They christened the vessel *Larooco* (rhymes with "cocoa"),[18] a portmanteau for Lawrence, Roosevelt, and Company. Franklin reprised his therapeutic cruises in the winters of 1924, 1925, and 1926 aboard what Lawrence dubbed their "floating tenement."[19]

Missy LeHand was the undisputed queen of the vessel, reigning over visits by family, friends, financiers, and high-powered politicians.[20] Missy shared a bond with Franklin that no other woman ever had. A bout with rheumatic fever at age fifteen had left her with its most dreaded aftermath—valvular heart disease which severely limited her capacity for physical activity.[21] Missy's ongoing battle with heart disease gave her an intimate understanding of the psychological consequences of Franklin's disability. During their months

---

16 McIntire, R., *White House Physician*. New York: G. P. Putnam's Sons, 1946, 30–34.
17 *Ibid*.
18 Roosevelt and Brough, 158.
19 Ward, *FCT*, 626.
20 Among them were businessman J.C Penney and Franklin's former running mate, James Cox.
21 Smith, K., 7.

alone together, she bore witness to demons no other person was permitted to see. "There were days on the *Larooco* when it was noon before he was able to pull himself out of depression and greet his guests wearing his lighthearted façade," Missy later confided to Frances Perkins.[22]

By 1926, Franklin was touting a miraculous recovery. A handwritten letter of March 26 bragged, "I am down here on a small boat & the legs are greatly improved—I get around now with no brace on right knee & hope to get rid of the other this summer."[23] It wasn't true then nor would it ever be.

Elliott Roosevelt recalled witnessing the intimacy between his father and Missy aboard *Larooco* as a young teenager. "Everyone in the closely-knit circle of father's friends accepted it as a matter of course," he later wrote. "I remember being only mildly stirred to see him with Missy in his lap ... holding her in his sun-browned arms whose clasp we children knew so well ... It was no great shock to discover that Missy had a familial life in all its aspects with father. What did surprise us was the later knowledge that mother knew too and accepted it as a fact of life like the rest of us."[24] The polio virus should not affect sexual function other than the ability to move muscles. A urinalysis of Fred Rosen, one of Franklin's aliases, on August 13, 1936, reveals the presence of "numerous motile organisms"—in other words, sperm—proof positive that Franklin was sexually active.[25]

At the other extreme, biographer and fellow polio victim Hugh Gallagher postulated in the 1980s that Franklin was celibate after contracting polio. He described Franklin's relationship with Missy as "his closest, his most intimate, to the last unconsummated ... Missy was, indeed, the lover who was not his lover."[26] The truth of the relationship will never be known; however, it is well known both Franklin and Missy had other romantic relationships.[27]

---

22 Ward, *FCT*, 696–697.
23 Collection of the author.
24 Roosevelt and Brough, 205. Elliott's comments seem plausible but cannot be taken at face value. His revelations about his father and Missy have been disputed by two of his brothers and his sister. Elliott became the black sheep of the family as a consequence of his numerous financially motivated exploitations of his parents' name and reputations.
25 Anna Halsted files, FDRL. Sperm appears in the urine in a condition known as retrograde ejaculation. Elliott asserted his father showed no evidence of *incontinentia coendi* (*Ibid.*, 198), as did a panel of doctors who examined him in 1930. While polio devastates muscles, it has no direct effect on sexual function.
26 Gallagher, 140.
27 Missy has been linked romantically to New York State policeman Earl Miller (as was Eleanor), as well as a long, well-documented relationship with Ambassador William

After her break with Franklin in 1918, Eleanor became comfortable with Missy's ability to provide her husband with the emotional support she was incapable of giving him. Missy's constant presence also relieved Eleanor of some of the ceremonial duties of a political spouse, freeing her to pursue her own personal and professional passions. Her alliance with Louis Howe had borne additional fruit. Under his tutelage, she overcame her fear of public speaking. He taught her to shed the nervous giggle of her girlhood and pitch her voice to a lower, more pleasant tone. Using her newfound associations with free-thinking, progressive women such as union leader Esther Schneiderman and Democratic leaders Esther Lape and her partner, Elizabeth Reed, Eleanor began speaking to feminist, labor, civic, and political groups, and became a force of her own. The strangest of bedfellows, Howe and Eleanor remained close until his death in April, 1936.[28]

Among the rotating cast of passengers aboard *Larooco* during its 1924 maiden voyage was James Cox, who urged his former running mate to reenter politics. New York Governor Alfred E. Smith was vying for the Democratic nomination for president that year and Cox suggested Franklin chair Smith's campaign. Smith took the prospect a step further, asking Franklin to nominate him at the Democratic convention, to be held in Manhattan's Madison Square Garden that June. Franklin was hesitant—he had not appeared in public since being stricken. But Eleanor, Louis, and Missy encouraged him to accept. He did, with the proviso that every effort be made to avoid revealing his infirmity.

Franklin's starring role in that act posed towering challenges. He had plenty of upper body strength, but in order to deliver the speech he had to get from his seat in the New York delegation to the podium under a reasonable facsimile of his own power. Taking that dare, Franklin devised a way to imitate walking by thrusting his paralyzed legs, stiffened with braces, from side to side as he gripped a crutch with his right hand, while tightly grasping the arm of his sixteen-year-old son James with his left. As they neared the lectern, James would step away and Franklin would take up a second crutch to cover the remaining distance. Rehearsing the routine, Franklin and James exhausted themselves

---

Bullitt. FDR had a strong emotional relationship with Margaret Suckley, Princess Martha of Norway, and possibly a physical one with New York *Post* publisher Dorothy Schiff. FDR and Missy's relationship evolved into that of an older brother/younger sister.

28 Some historians believe Eleanor's personal relationship with Howe was closer than it was with Franklin. Eleanor, for instance arranged for Howe's White House funeral. See: Petrusza, D., *Roosevelt Sweeps Nation: FDR's 1936 Landslide & the Triumph of the Liberal Ideal*. New York: Diversion Books, 2022, Chapter 2.

marching back and forth in the library and hallway of their East 65th Street townhouse.

Franklin's nominating speech was written by a Smith aide, New York State Supreme Court Justice Joseph Proskauer. For the first time, a nationwide radio audience was tuned in to a political convention. As 8,000 delegates, alternates, and spectators, including Sara, Eleanor, and his four oldest children, held their collective breath, Franklin let go of James's arm, muscled himself to the specially constructed lectern, and firmly grasped the handholds. He threw back his head and flashed his trademark smile—earning a three-minute round of applause. His thirty-four-minute oration closed with a sentence that entered history: "He is the 'Happy Warrior' of the political battlefield—Alfred E. Smith!"[29] The delegates gave Franklin another uproarious standing ovation. According to the head of the Missouri delegation Tom Prendergast, had Franklin "been physically able to withstand the campaign, he would have been nominated by acclamation."[30] From that point on, Franklin was back as a serious political presence.

The nominating speech was the high point of the convention for Smith. His quest for the Democratic nod came up against the Ku Klux Klan, then at the zenith of its political power and unwilling to permit a Catholic nominee, no less one who opposed Prohibition. After seventeen days and 102 ballots in stifling heat, exhausted delegates nominated a weak compromise candidate, West Virginia attorney John W. Davis. Wilson's former Solicitor General and ambassador to England went on to take 28.8 percent of the popular vote—closer to the 16.6 of Wisconsin Progressive Robert La Follette, than the victor Calvin Coolidge's 54.

---

29 FDR didn't like the speech, telling Proskauer, "It will probably be a flop." Judge Joseph Proskauer Interview, Columbia Oral History Project, Columbia University.
30 Dunlap, I.B., *FDR*, July 10, 1924, quoted in Smith, J.E., *Ibid.*, 212.

Chapter 7
Old Doctor Roosevelt

At the Madison Square Garden Democratic convention, Franklin ran into banker, philanthropist, and party kingpin George Foster Peabody, who crowed about his recent purchase of a rundown hotel and health spa in the remote Georgia village of Bullochville and his hopes of reinvigorating the operation.[1] The resort's draw was a natural warm spring whose mineral waters had been touted since Civil War times as beneficial for a variety of ailments. Peabody followed up the meeting with a letter that included a testimonial by Louis Joseph, a seven-year-old polio victim who claimed he had regained his ability to walk after bathing in the spa's waters.[2] The notion of therapeutic mineral waters resonated with Franklin's boyhood memories of the spa at Bad Nauheim. He agreed to visit Bullochville after Tom Loyless, Peabody's partner in the venture, made a visit to New York to solicit his participation.[3]

On October 3, 1924, Franklin, Eleanor, Missy, and Leroy Jones were met at the Bullochville train station by fifty of the town's 470 residents and driven to a ramshackle cottage deep in a pine forest. The next morning, Peabody and Loyless delivered the storied Louis Joseph to the cottage and gave their honored guests a tour of the town. Franklin was focused on the therapeutic waters and looked beyond the rickety three-story Meriwether Inn and the dilapidated cottages adjacent to it. Missy, who had come along to handle Franklin's business correspondence, had been raised in a blue-collar Boston suburb and enjoyed the rustic local color and the magnificent vistas from Pine Mountain. Eleanor was repulsed by the squalor of Jim Crow Georgia and caught the next train back to New York.

Franklin's first swim in the spa's pool was enthralling. The buoyancy of the mineral water permitted him to stand chest deep. For the first time in three years, he was able to move his toes. He and Missy remained in Georgia for a month to complete a course of therapy.

---

1 The nearest paved road was ten miles away.
2 Steven, R., *Hi-Ya Neighbor*. New York and Atlanta: Tupper and Love, 1947, 3.
3 Ward, *FCT*, 702–703.

Peabody and Loyless had convinced town leaders to rename Bullochville as "Warm Springs" and asked Franklin to give a speech to commemorate the occasion. He used the opportunity to laud the waters' benefits based on personal experience. An *Atlanta Journal* reporter wrote up the event for his newspaper's Sunday supplement and editors across the nation reprinted "Franklin D. Roosevelt Will Swim to Health."

By the time Franklin returned for another round of treatment in March 1925, polio victims, "polios" as they were simply called, and their families were making medical pilgrimages to the resort. Never missing an opportunity to ingratiate himself, Franklin assumed the role of informal host—organizing picnics, card games, and other activities. He also performed detailed physical examinations of fellow patients and used his considerable self-taught knowledge of therapeutic techniques to treat them. Franklin's evaluations of muscle strength were as accurate as any physician's today. He came to be known around town as "Old Doctor Roosevelt," a moniker he did not discourage. The title was appropriate. Despite his lack of formal medical training, Franklin was among his era's most innovative and effective rehabilitative clinicians.

Equally important, Franklin understood polio's deep psychological impact. As Geoffrey C. Ward, himself a polio victim, noted, "Roosevelt did not invent physiotherapy, of course, but he was an authentic pioneer in its application, and his eager, infectious enthusiasm galvanized 'polios' who until they met him had been utterly without hope." Polios often seemed addled when they got to Warm Springs, one of the resort's first physiotherapists later remembered, "The impact of the disease was so devastating, both for them and their families, that they no longer knew who they were or why they were. At Warm Springs they found out."[4]

In July 1925, Dr. Draper wrote to Franklin to ask if he would be willing to donate blood serum for an early attempt at immunotherapy for polio.[5]

"Dear Franklin,

"Would you consider letting me take some blood from you in order to make serum to treat acute cases of infantile paralysis? The miserable disease is beginning to show itself again around these parts and I should like to have

4 *Ibid.*, 723.
5 Treatment with immune serum continues to be utilized, as recently witnessed during the 2019/2020 pandemic of COVID-19.

some serum on hand. I could take about 500 cubic centimeters [roughly 17 ounces] from you, which I do not think you will notice at all. And that would be enough to treat two cases."[6] Franklin's reply was gracious and humorous.

"Dear George,

"Sure, you can bleed me. You have not bled me as much as some other doctors, so you are entitled to the opportunity ... How many cocktails does one need after the bloodletting to restore the circulation?"[7]

Against the admonishments of family and friends, Franklin bought the resort on April 26, 1926. The final cost of the complicated deal was $200,000 (more than $3,500,000 in 2022), about two-thirds of his available assets, for title to the springs themselves, the Meriwether Inn, thirteen ramshackle cottages, and 1,100 acres.[8]

For the first time in his life, Franklin had total control of a business and jumped in with manic enthusiasm, laying out plans for refurbishing the pools and building cottages for year-round use. "I am consulting architect and landscaping engineer for the Warm Springs Co.," he wrote to his Harvard pal Livy Davis, "... am giving advice on the moving of buildings, the building of roads, setting out of trees, and remodeling the hotel ... a new water system, new sewage plant, fishing pond, golf course and other forms of indoor and outdoor sports." Franklin recruited physicians, nurses, and "physios," as physical therapists were known at the time.

All this enterprise required money. Franklin and Basil "Doc" O'Connor his law partner since New Year's day 1925, who would become a lifelong intimate confidant, created the charitable Warm Springs Foundation, so affluent friends and business connections might derive tax benefits from their donations.[9] Prominent contributors included automobile magnate Edsel Ford. Vincent Astor's wife, Helen, was appointed to the Board of Directors.

Old Doctor Roosevelt's empathy extended beyond polio patients. Missy LeHand's heart condition had rendered her prone to episodes of atrial fibrillation, a disconnection between the heart's pumping chambers that sapped her

---

6 Draper to FDR, July 23, 1925, FDRL.
7 FDR to Draper, July 25, 1925, FDRL.
8 Tobin, 219.
9 Rose, D.W., *Friends and Partners.* Amsterdam: Academic Press (Elsevier), 2016, 43.

stamina. The one effective treatment was foxglove, a medicinal plant known to doctors by its scientific name, digitalis.[10] A side effect of the drug often sent Missy into weeks of delirium. Her health had been poor during the last half of 1927 so Franklin arranged for a recuperative stay at Warm Springs. "The child has been much more seriously ill last summer than she realizes," he wrote to Missy's Aunt Nellie, "and though she is so much better now, it is most important for her to keep very quiet and avoid colds and excitement during this winter."[11]

Franklin strived to gain the endorsement of the mainstream medical community, but was repeatedly and discourteously snubbed. Once again in the role of underdog, he found an ally in Boston, Dr. Robert Osgood, who had taken over Dr. Lovett's orthopedic practice.[12] Osgood helped Franklin recruit Dr. Leroy Hubbard, retired chief of the New York State Public Health Service, who brought along his able physio, Helena Maloney. Those affiliations helped give Warm Springs the credibility it lacked. Still, Franklin was labeled a quack and a profiteer. In February 1928, he sent an angry letter to Morris Fishbein, the very influential editor of the *Journal of the American Medical Association*.

"The trustees of the Georgia Warm Springs Foundation and Dr. Hubbard, the Surgeon in Chief, are leaning over backwards to conform strictly to what you gentlemen call 'medical ethics," Franklin wrote to Fishbein. "There are undoubtedly many people in the medical profession who have not believed the great strides in the past two or three years in results obtained from giving directed exercises in the medium of warm water for infantile paralysis cases ... no claims of cure-all or exaggerated results have been made, are being made or will be made." A handwritten postscript added, "My only kick is about your telling people that advertising literature was being circulated for the 'resort' and that the 'thing' was evidently 'a kind of promotion'—of course none of these things happen to be true!"[13]

---

10 The therapeutic benefits of digitalis, also known as Foxglove, were first described by English physician and botanist William Withering in 1785.
11 FDR to Nellie Graffin. December 29, 1927 collection of the author.
12 Tobin, 192.
13 FDR to Dr. Morris Fishbein, February 20, 1928. Collection of the author.

◼ Chapter 8
◼ Back in the Game

Franklin's oratory at the 1924 Democratic convention had reinstated him in the national political conversation. The only uncertainty was when, rather than if, he would pursue elected office. He declined an invitation to run for United States Senate in 1926, pleading the necessity for more time to recover from polio. In truth, he was not yet ready to confront the rigors of public life and didn't want the job anyway. In 1928, Al Smith, now the front-runner for the Democratic presidential nomination, asked Franklin to nominate him for a second time. Unlike four years earlier, FDR wrote his own speech. The effect on delegates in Houston was even more electrifying than 1924. "It is seldom that a political speech attains this kind of eloquence," *The New York Times* wrote, calling the address "a model of its kind."[1]

Not only did Franklin impress conventioneers, he specifically targeted his message for fifteen million radio listeners nationwide. "I tried the experiment of writing and delivering my speech wholly for the benefit of the radio audience and the press," he wrote to journalist Walter Lippmann. "Smith had the votes anyway and it seemed to me more important to reach out for the Republicans and independents throughout the country."[2] It was a transformational moment in FDR's political career. His remarkable rhetorical skills were a perfect fit for the powerful new medium of radio. From this point on, the only contacts the vast majority of the American public had with him was what they heard in their living rooms, read in magazines and local newspapers, or saw in newsreels and carefully edited photographs.

Franklin's surging popularity led Smith to press him to run for Governor of New York in the belief that he was the one Democrat capable of holding the statehouse and carrying the state for Smith against a strong GOP nominee, New York State Attorney General Albert Ottinger. Franklin declined at first, citing his finances and his all-encompassing involvement with Warm Springs. But Smith's campaign manager, John J. Raskob, who held top financial positions at both DuPont and General Motors, jumped in to nullify those concerns

---

1 *New York Times*, June 28, 1928.
2 Smith, J.E., 313.

by promising to underwrite Franklin's expenses in Georgia.[3] Over the next four years, Raskob was the Warm Springs Foundation's leading benefactor.[4]

Franklin accepted the nomination for governor over the vigorous objection of Missy LeHand, by now his most significant social and professional female relationship. From 1925 through 1928, he was away from home 116 out of 208 weeks. Eleanor was with him for four, his mother for two—and Missy for 110.[5]

The decision to run for governor forced Franklin to come to grips with the fact that his days of total dedication to recovery from polio were over. Nonetheless, many news articles were portraying him as having made a near-total recovery. Typical was a 1927 report he had "discarded the crutches" he had needed at the 1924 convention and "a brace and a cane is all he needs to lead his active life."[6] Franklin doubled down. "Seven years ago, in the epidemic in New York, I came down with infantile paralysis, a perfectly normal attack, and I was completely, for the moment, put out of my useful activities. By personal good fortune, I was able to get the very best of care, and the result … is that today I am on my feet."[7]

A gubernatorial campaign presented physical challenges for a wheelchair-bound candidate, especially one intent on concealing his disability. "He could not climb stairs, and often we had to carry him up some backstairs to a hall and down again," speechwriter Sam Rosenman recalled. "He always went through this harrowing experience smiling. He never got ruffled. Having been set down, he would adjust his coat, smile and proceed calmly to the platform for his speech."[8]

---

3 Raskob worked his way up at DuPont to become its chief financial officer in 1918. He orchestrated DuPont's large minority share in General Motors and created the General Motors Assistance Program (GMAC), which enabled dealers to offer their customers credit for installment payments. After a political dispute with Alfred P. Sloan, GM's Republican CEO, Raskob sold his GM stock and used the money to finance construction of the Empire State Building. A close ally of Smith, he became DNC chairman in 1928 and resigned in 1932. After Smith broke with FDR, Raskob joined him in opposition to Roosevelt's "liberal" New Deal policies.

4 Friedel, 255.

5 Ward, *FCT*, 709.

6 Unidentified clipping in Paul Hasbrouck file, FDRL-HP, quoted in Houck, D.W., Kiewe, A.., *FDR's Body Politics*, College Station: Texas A & M University Press, 2003, xii,141.

7 Gilbert, R.E., *The Mortal Presidency*. New York: Fordham University Press, 1998, 47.

8 Rosenman, S., *Working with Roosevelt*. New York: Harper & Brothers, 1952, 22.

New York Republicans brought up the health issue. "There is something both pathetic and pitiless in the 'drafting' of Franklin D. Roosevelt," asserted the *New York Post*. "The nomination is unfair to Mr. Roosevelt and it is equally unfair to the people of the state," said the *Herald Tribune*. "A governor doesn't have to be an acrobat," Al Smith responded. "The work of the governorship is brainwork. Frank Roosevelt is mentally as good as he ever was in his life."[9],[10]

"No movies of me getting out of the machine, boys," Franklin told photographers as he arrived at the Hyde Park polling station on Election Day. The cameramen paused their work until he had been lifted from his seat and his braces had been snapped into position. Once hoisted from the car, he posed for photos.[11] News photographers "voluntarily destroyed their own plates [if] they showed Roosevelt in poses that revealed his handicap."[12] Other photographs were staged and retouched to leave the impression Franklin could stand without assistance. This code of silence was never broken in FDR's lifetime.

Hoover soundly defeated Smith on November 6, 1928, but Franklin took the New York governorship by a little over 25,000 of more than 4,000,000 votes cast. The winning margin came from Republican districts upstate and was not recorded until the next morning. Even before election officials certified victory, Franklin left for a month in Warm Springs, "resting and taking treatments there" so as to be "in fit condition to assume the duties of Chief Executive." *The New York Times* declared him "the heir apparent to the leadership of the Democratic Party."[13]

Franklin promptly distanced himself from Smith and his key aides, Belle Moskowitz and Robert Moses, making it clear that the former three-time Governor was not going to be running the incoming administration from the sidelines. Relations between FDR and Smith cooled. Still, Franklin had inherited a well-run government and enjoyed a smooth transition to his new administration.

As governor, Franklin perfected the use of chatty radio addresses to keep in touch with New Yorkers. As a consequence, legislators were deluged with

---

9 Lindley, E.K., *Franklin D. Roosevelt, A Career in Progressive Democracy*. Indianapolis, IN: Bobbs Merrill, 1931, 41.

10 Smith, J.E., 317.

11 Winfield, B.H., *FDR and the News Media*. New York: Columbia University Press, 1994, 16.

12 *Ibid*., quoting Leuchtenberg, W., *FDR and the New Deal*. New York: Harper Perenniel, 2009

13 *New York Times*, November 11, 1928.

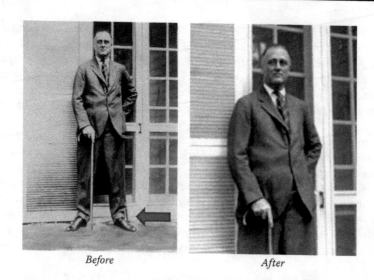

Before   *After*

letters in support of his progressive agenda. When Wall Street crashed in late 1929, he was among the first state chief executives to support farmers with government subsidies and to take action against rising unemployment.[14]

Despite a successful two-year term as governor, Franklin's health was still an issue during the 1930 reelection campaign. On October 18, with three weeks remaining, Dr. E.W. Beckwith, medical director of the Equitable Life Assurance Society, announced at a press conference in Albany that Equitable and twenty-one other companies had agreed to insure Franklin's life for $560,000 ($10,000,000 in 2022) payable to the Warm Springs Foundation. "It has rarely been my privilege to see such a remarkable physical specimen as yourself," Beckwith declared, "and I trust that your remarkable vitality will stand you in good stead throughout your arduous campaign." The doctor announced that the 48-year-old governor's "examination disclosed conditions which were comparable to a man of thirty," including a blood pressure of 128/82. "Given the exam took place the same week as the Democratic state convention," said Beckwith, "he has been under very great strain, and it was an astonishing fact that his heart and blood pressure were absolutely normal, and he passed an unusually good examination for a man who has just been through such a trying ordeal." When asked about Franklin's paralysis, Beckwith responded, "Frankly, I have never before observed such a complete degree of recovery in organic function and such a remarkable degree

---

14 Smith, J.E., 242.

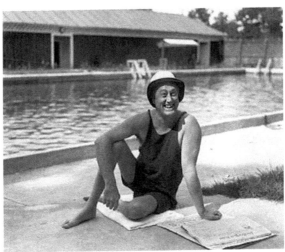

FDR at Warm Springs 1924 showing marked leg atrophy

of recovery of muscles and limbs in an individual who has passed through an attack of infantile paralysis such as yours."[15]

Franklin boasted he kept fit with daily swims and horseback riding—the latter an impossibility for a person with virtually no functioning leg muscles. "I watch my weight carefully," he said. "I don't want to weigh more than 175 pounds." At the time he was tipping the scales at 182.[16]

Franklin coasted to reelection by 735,000 votes. The previously highest plurality had been 386,000 for Smith in 1922.[17] "It was not the depression that brought the extraordinary victory, for there was no similar Democratic trend that year in the New York Congressional elections," speechwriter Sam Rosenman noted. "It was the warmth of Roosevelt the man and the orator, who knew how to convey his personality and charm to the people he met and to the people he talked with over the air."[18] Campaign manager James A. Farley told reporters, "I do not see how Mr. Roosevelt can escape becoming the next presidential candidate."

---

15 *New York Times*, October, 19, 1930.
16 Smith, J.E., 244.
17 Rosenman, 47.
18 *Ibid.*

Louis Howe sent angry rebuttals to newspapers that questioned Franklin's physical fitness. Beckwith's report had given him ammunition, as had another examination conducted two months later. The ploy was orchestrated by Earl Looker, a freelance writer with connections to the Republican Roosevelts. In December 1930, Looker informed Eleanor of his intention to write a book about Franklin to be published in time for the 1932 presidential campaign, telling her he had the support of powerful unidentified backers. Looker's anonymous angels were the editors of the Democratic-leaning magazine *Liberty*, America's highest-circulation weekly.

Looker proposed that Franklin undergo a full medical examination. The candidate responded on February 23, 1931, offering his complete cooperation. An elite, independent panel composed of Samuel W. Lambert, former dean of Columbia University's College of Physicians and Surgeons, orthopedist Russell A. Hibbs, and Foster Kennedy, chief neurologist at Bellevue Hospital, examined Franklin on April 29. Their findings were published in the July 25 issue of *Liberty* under the headline "Is Franklin D. Roosevelt Physically Fit to Be President?" The article included two photos never published again in Franklin's lifetime—one showing him seated in his office with his leg braces visible; the other poolside in a bathing suit at Warm Springs in 1924, his atrophied legs in plain view.[19]

The surprisingly candid piece conceded that "[Franklin's] legs [are] not much good to him," but the doctors' conclusion about the question of fitness to serve was a resounding "yes." Dr. Lambert, a Republican, later qualified his endorsement: "As far as I'm concerned, this doesn't go for above the neck."[20]

Even before the issue hit the newsstands, Louis Howe had sent thousands of copies to journalists and Democratic officials, reminding them that a trio of distinguished doctors had pronounced Franklin's "lameness" to be "steadily getting better," and how he "can walk all necessary distances and can maintain a standing position without fatigue."[21,22] "Well, Sir, we got away with the *Liberty* article, despite all obstacles." Looker wrote to Franklin, "At least seven

---

19 *Liberty*, July 25, 1931.

20 Krock, A., *Sixty Years on the Firing Line*. New York: Funk and Wagnall's, 1968, 152. As quoted in Lomazow and Fettmann, 46.

21 *New York Times*, July 1, 1932.

22 Unlike the insurance exam six months earlier, the doctors Looker hired did not release specific findings, which did not become public until five years after Roosevelt's death. Franklin's blood pressure was 140/100, a significant elevation over his 128/82 from the previous October (a normal level for a man of forty-nine was 120/80).

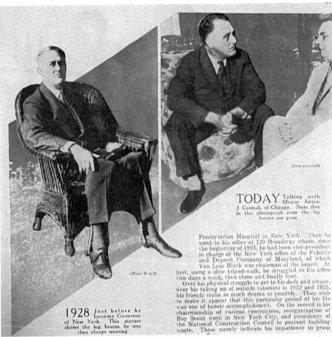

Photos from article in Physical Culture, April 1932, minimizing the appearance of FDR's braces.

and a half million readers are sure you are physically fit!"[23] Jim Farley pronounced the article "a corker." Franklin's polio "had no more effect on his general condition than if he had a glass eye or was prematurely bald," Farley said.[24]

When an enthusiastic supporter sent Franklin a biography he intended to publish that mentioned he "suffered" from polio, Governor Roosevelt shot back a reply on July 9, 1931. "This is the first chance I have had to thank you for your letter and to read it over. I have made a number of corrections as to the facts. By the way, I don't 'suffer.' I have no pain and except for a weak knee muscle, [I'm] probably in better health than ninety nine people out of a hundred."[25]

---

23 Lomazow and Fettmann, 47. Quoted from Houck and Kiewe, 70.
24 Neal, S., *Happy Days are Here Again: The 1932 Convention, the Emergence of FDR—and How America Was Changed Forever.* New York: Harper Collins, 2004, 175.
25 FDR to Joseph Lieb, July 9, 1931. Private collection.

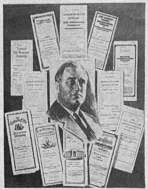

Half a Million Life Insurance

Twenty-two life insurance companies, less than two years ago, underwrote $500,000 life insurance for Franklin D. Roosevelt. No physical tests are more searching than life insurance examinations on which money is risked. They found that

Franklin D. Roosevelt is sound, healthy and physically fit.

Three eminent doctors, Dr. Samuel W. Lambert, outstanding diagnostician; the late Russell A. Hibbs, chief surgeon of the New York Orthopedic Dispensary and Hospital, and Dr. Foster Kennedy, nerve specialist, examined Franklin D. Roosevelt last year at the request of *Liberty Magazine.* They reported:

Franklin D. Roosevelt's health and powers of endurance are such as to allow him to meet any demand of private and public life.

Twelve years ago Franklin D. Roosevelt suffered an attack of infantile paralysis. Today he is fully recovered except that his legs are partially disabled. For four years, as Governor of New York, he has worked tirelessly, early and late, for the people of his state. In this presidential campaign he has made a strenuous cross-country tour that would exhaust the ordinary person. Franklin D. Roosevelt's magnificent and victorious fight against the handicap of a dread disease is another proof—perhaps the most dramatic—of his grit, his courage, his strength of character.

Stop the Whispering Campaign
Elect a Strong Leader — FRANKLIN D. ROOSEVELT

Issued by the Democratic National Campaign Committee
Hotel Biltmore—New York City

Campaign ad for FDR's 1932 presidential campaign.

Another Looker article in April 1932 in health guru Bernarr MacFadden's *Physical Culture* magazine attempted to create the impression that Franklin did not need braces at all![26]

As planned, Looker expanded the *Liberty* article into *This Man Roosevelt*, a 1932 campaign biography that cast Franklin's health in glowing terms. "I walked with him many times from the entrance hall into the Capitol, some fifty paces," Looker wrote. "Walking some twenty paces more from the desk, he eases himself into his big Governor's chair and flexes his leg braces so that his knees bend under the edge of his desk. He seems unfatigued. In fact the only reason for his braces is to insure his knees locking."[27] Looker's exercise in political propaganda went a long way toward discrediting whispers about Franklin's health.

With a depression raging, President Hoover insisted that direct relief for unemployment distress was not a federal responsibility—no matter the cost in human misery. Hoover's remedy was to offer loans to railroads, financial institutions, and other large corporations. In stark contrast, Franklin had delivered his "What is the State?" speech to an emergency session of the New York State legislature on August 28, 1931.[28] The address boldly asserted that the state had a "social duty" to care for those who cannot care for themselves. Legislators enacted the Temporary Emergency Relief Administration (TERA), funded by $23,000,000 in new taxes ($450,000,000 in 2022).[29] A three-man board led by Jesse Strauss, president of the R.H. Macy retail chain, chose Iowan Harry Hopkins to be TERA's executive director. Hopkins, president of the National Association of Social Workers, had vast experience in child welfare and public health. TERA furnished direct aid to 1.2 million New Yorkers "to provide them with food, clothing and shelter" and put 80,000 more to work with $5,000,000 ($98,000,000 in 2022) allocated for work relief programs.[30,31]

26 Looker, E., "Franklin Roosevelt's Come-Back from Invalidism." *Physical Culture* April 1932;47(4):17–19, 55–57.

27 Looker, E., *This Man Roosevelt*. New York: Brewer, Warren and Putnam, 1932, 147. Quoted in Houck and Kiewe, 74.

28 Rosenman, 50.

29 Roll, D., *The Hopkins Touch*. OUP, 2013, 227.

30 Rosenman, 52.

31 See: https://www.encyclopedia.com/economics/encyclopedias-almanacs-transcripts-and-maps/temporary-emergency-relief-administration-new-york-tera.

After Franklin announced his candidacy for the presidency on January 22, 1932, Sam Rosenman told him, "If you were nominated tomorrow it would be pretty hard to get up intelligent speeches overnight on the many subjects you would have to discuss." Rosenman argued against relying for advice on the usual band of industrialists, financiers, and national political leaders. "Why not go to the universities of the country?" he suggested. "They wouldn't be afraid to strike out on new paths."[32] Thus was born a new concept in political jargon, the "brain trust."

The key original member of Franklin's brain trust was Raymond Moley, a Columbia University professor, political economist, and executive director of Franklin's New York State Commission on the Administration of Justice. "He believes in your social philosophy and objectives and has a clear and force-ful style of writing," Rosenman told Franklin.[33] Moley recruited like-minded Columbia colleagues, among them economist Rexford Tugwell, a strong advo-cate for governmental control of economic matters, and Adolf A. Berle, co-au-thor of a treatise regarding the foundations of United States corporate law.

On April 7, 1932, Franklin delivered his manifesto in a radio address, now known as the "forgotten man" speech, written in large part by Moley. "These unhappy times," Franklin told the American people, "call for the building of plans that rest upon the forgotten, the unorganized but the indispensable units of economic power, for plans that build from the bottom up and not from the top down, that put their faith once more in the forgotten man at the bottom of the economic pyramid."

---

32 Rosenman, 57.
33 This was true at the time, but Moley later broke with Franklin over his economic policy and by 1940 became a conservative Republican.

■ Chapter 9
■ The Nourmahal Gang

A photograph of Franklin on the cover of the May 28, 1923, issue of *Time* shows a seemingly inconsequential triangular-shaped pigmentation above his left eyebrow, known to dermatologists as a macule.[1,2] Franklin spent the next six years baking in sunlight as an integral part of his polio recovery regimen. By 1930, the forehead freckle had enlarged and darkened, taking on the appearance of a highly malignant cancer then erroneously classified as melanotic sarcoma, now simply called melanoma.

Medical science had not yet connected the relationship between melanoma and exposure of the skin to ultraviolet radiation in sunlight, but doctors at the time were well aware of how deadly the cancer was. A review of the contemporary medical literature reveals the prognosis and state-of-the-art treatment for melanoma in the early 1930s:

> "Melanotic sarcoma is highly malignant and almost invariably fatal, but in some cases the patient can lead a normal life for up to twelve years."[3,4]

> "Optimal treatment is a wide surgical excision of the primary lesion and/or radiation with high-voltage x-ray or radium."[5]

---

1 *Time,* May 28, 1923. The photograph traced to an article about FDR's role as president of the American Construction Council and declared—at best, grossly misleading; at worst, flatly untrue—that "he is no longer an invalid."

2 Williams, G., Karcher, M., "Nomenclature of Skin Lesions," www.pediatrics.wisc.edu/education/derm.text.html.

3 Dwight Wilbur and Howard Hartman of the Mayo Clinic wrote in 1931: "Malignant melanoma, frequently termed melanosarcoma or melano-epithelioma, is one of the most malignant tumors encountered in man. In some instances, however, the body seems to possess unusual resistance to metastasis from these tumors and it may be years after the appearance or removal of the primary growth before sudden, rapid and overwhelming metastasis occurs."

4 Handley, S. summarized in the June 15, 1935, issue of *The Lancet:* "It is customary to speak of melanotic sarcoma as the most malignant of known tumors. It is certainly not the most rapidly fatal. The average duration of a case of melanotic sarcoma is three years and up to within months of the end the patient remains free from pain and able to get about." Handley wrote.

5 A 1932 article by Hubert J. Farrell of the Mayo Clinic was similarly bleak: "the prognosis in cases of melanoma is more unfavorable than that of any other type of malignant neoplasm

Franklin and his physicians confronted a Hobson's choice. The best chance for a cure was the most aggressive—removing as much of the tumor as possible along with a considerable volume of surrounding bone and soft tissue, coupled with intensive irradiation. This would have been the course of action had Franklin's growth been on his torso or a limb, but taking that approach above an eye would have inflicted horrific disfigurement, inevitably signaling that he had cancer and putting an abrupt end to his life in politics. Instead, it was decided to treat the tumor as aggressively as possible while camouflaging its existence—the beginning of an ultra-secret deception that persisted for the remainder of his life.

In 1927, Vincent Astor had commissioned a 264-foot steel yacht to be built by renowned shipbuilders Friedrich Krupp Germaniawerft, who had built the German war fleet. He spent a year in Kiel, Germany, overseeing his behemoth's construction.[6] *Nourmahal*, named in memory of a yacht beloved by Vincent's late father, had a crew of forty-two and conservatively cost $100,000 a year ($1,700,000 in 2022) to maintain. The world's most luxurious private yacht had nine staterooms, eight bathrooms, a fully equipped sick bay, and a cruising range of 12,000 miles.

An introvert by nature, Vincent used *Nourmahal* to escape from the press. "Mr. Astor discovered early the solace of the sea," *Time* wrote on February 6, 1928. "Reporters cannot infest the oceans. The strain of question and answer to which a public figure is eternally subjected is particularly distasteful to the new commodore. Once, shrewdly said he: 'The social gulf between Americans is not so much measured in money as in newspaper headlines.'" Franklin had similar sentiments, referring to his cruises, including those aboard

---

... the outlook in late cases of melanoma is very poor in any event, and rather than subject the patient to radical surgical procedures it would probably be better to vie intensive roentgenologic treatment as a palliative measure ... In spite of the high degree of malignancy, and the rapid onset of death following dissemination of metastatic growth, some persons seem to possess unusual resistance to invasion of the internal organs by these growths. It is probable that metastasis has already taken place at the time of excision of the primary growth but many years may elapse before death occurs. There were nine cases in this series and the interval between the time of excision varied from five to twelve years ... Lesions should be radically excised early. About 4 cm of normal skin on all sides should be included, and the incision should be deep enough to include subcutaneous tissue. Early radical removal of any type of nevus subjected to trauma is the only means of reducing the high mortality rates of melanomas." Cutaneous Melanomas with Special Reference to Prognosis *Arch Derm Syph* 1932;25:110–124.

6 Germany had been banned from producing warships by the Treaty of Versailles.

Nourmahal, as "the only place I can get away from people, telephones, and uniforms."[7]

An elite group of Astor's friends, which included Franklin, came to be known as the "*Nourmahal* Gang," named for their regular excursions aboard the pleasure craft.[8] The group comprised of gentry with whom Astor was socially comfortable. He treated these elite shipmates to scientific expeditions to the Galapagos Islands and world tours spiced with fishing, gambling, and carousing.

In 1931, the *Nourmahal* Gang acquired a new member with a background starkly different from the group's privileged profile. Dr. W. Leslie Heiter, the son of a print-shop owner, was a native of Mobile, Alabama, who had received his medical degree from Tulane University in 1928. Dr. Heiter came to New York City in June 1929 for a six-month internship at America's most prestigious cancer treatment center, the Memorial Hospital for the Treatment of Cancer and Allied Diseases.[9] During his training at Memorial, Dr. Heiter reported his successful surgical treatment of "a case of unusual sinus involvement" during the hospital's weekly cancer conference and followed with a paper entitled "A Case of Carcinoma [cancer] of the Nasal Mucosa with Extension to the Frontal Sinus" in its journal. The article's publication was testimony to Heiter's expertise in treating an unusual, highly malignant form of cancer. After completing his stint at Memorial, Heiter remained in Manhattan for a year, spending 1930 at Cornell Medical College's prestigious New York Hospital to gain additional experience as a surgeon. One of his patients there was a young heiress, Helen Hooper Brown.[10] Dr. Heiter's demeanor and skill

---

7 FDR Personal Letters, I, 394.

8 Vincent Astor emerged from the Great War with an interest in intelligence gathering had been slipping nuggets of intelligence concerning the Caribbean and Panama Canal Zone to FDR since 1933. He had also been using *Nourmahal* to surveil the western coast of South America. In 1927, Astor organized a cadre of powerful gentry who shared a common interest in espionage, national defense, and a robust economy into a secret fraternity he called "The Room." The group met monthly in a nondescript apartment at 34 East 62nd Street in Manhattan to discuss international social, military, and economic matters. "The Room" comprised of an aristocracy of wealth and power, including members of the "*Nourmahal* Gang," real estate mogul and renowned *bon vivant*, William Rhinelander Stewart Jr., reformist Judge Frederic Kernochan and Theodore Roosevelt's son, Kermit, as well as a physician, Dr. Eugene Hillhouse Pool, president of the New York Hospital medical staff, who, in 1930 was instrumental in recruiting a cancer surgeon for FDR.

9 Heiter papers, in the possession of Bill Heiter, Mobile, Alabama.

10 Helen Hooper's inheritance came from the shovel and railroad business of her mother's Ames family, equivalent to $300,000,000 in 2022.

so impressed her that she wrote him to say, "remember you have a friend who wants to help in any way she can."[11] Mrs. Brown was the wife of Lathrop Brown, Franklin's Groton classmate and Harvard roommate. In 1911, Franklin had been best man at the couple's wedding.

Dr. Heiter was introduced to Vincent Astor by surgeon Eugene Hillhouse Pool, president of New York Hospital's medical staff. Dr. Pool was Astor's personal physician, friend, and later a member of the *"Nourmahal* Gang."[12] He had recognized Heiter's considerable professional and social skills. Mrs. Brown was likely involved. Dr. Heiter wrote to his father that the heiress was "the professor's [Dr. Pool's] prize patient."[13] Through this chain of connections, Dr. Heiter was recruited to treat Governor Roosevelt's melanoma. The significance of the timeline cannot be overstated—*the doctor/ patient relationship between Franklin D. Roosevelt and cancer surgeon Dr. W. Leslie Heiter began in the latter half of 1930.*

Heiter and Astor became fast friends, a bond that persisted long after the doctor returned to Alabama in 1931 to establish his practice.[14] Heiter accepted invitations to cruise the Caribbean on *Nourmahal* that year and again in 1932 for a trip to the Galapagos Islands, the Marquesas Islands, and Tahiti.

---

11 Helen Hooper Brown to Dr. Heiter. Undated but written in the second half of 1930. Heiter papers.
12 Dr. Pool operated on Astor for acute appendicitis in late 1930. He was also a member of Astor's secret fraternity of gentry "The Room."
13 Heiter papers.
14 Heiter eventually settled into the practice of obstetrics.

■ Chapter 10
■ The Road to the White House

Leading up to the 1932 Democratic convention in Chicago, Republicans once again attacked Franklin by raising doubts about his physical fitness. The Hoover camp went so far as to circulate a rumor he had advanced syphilis.[1] The Democrats parried with rebuttals by political and medical surrogates.

Franklin had the support of a majority of committed delegates, but not the two-thirds needed for nomination. Embittered at being denied another try at the presidency, Al Smith mobilized a "Stop Roosevelt" campaign. Franklin's health was targeted again. Smith's surrogate, New Jersey political boss Frank Hague, asked, "Why consider the one man who is weakest in the eyes of the rank and file?"[2]

To counter the eleventh-hour insurgency, the Roosevelt camp offered the vice presidency to Speaker of the House, John Nance Garner, ensuring the support of his native Texas delegation as well as that of his acolyte, media mogul William Randolph Hearst. The campaign also gained the support of the California delegation by giving its leader, William G. McAdoo, veto power over cabinet choices at State and Treasury. These arrangements put Franklin over the top on the fourth ballot. In an unprecedented move, Franklin flew to Illinois to accept the nomination. His speech at Chicago Stadium electrified delegates and radio listeners alike, closing with the vow, "I pledge you, I pledge myself, to a New Deal for the American people."

Franklin conducted a vigorous eighteen-week, 25,000-mile whistle-stop campaign on a schedule intended to dispel any notion he was disabled. His opponent was shackled to the worsening economic depression. Displaced families were sheltering in makeshift shantytowns they labeled "Hoovervilles."

---

1 With just three weeks to go, Oklahoma governor "Alfalfa Bill" Murray asked, "How much less can a man think who has locomotor ataxia (a form of advanced syphilis), a nervous disease that affects the spinal column, and ultimately the brain? I know they say it is infantile paralysis, but locomotor ataxia never came from that source."

2 Neal, 174.

Hoover was also stung by another publicity disaster. In 1924, Congress had awarded World War I veterans a $1,000 ($17,500 in 2022) bonus redeemable in 1945. In August 1932, fifteen thousand financially strapped former dough-boys, some with their families in tow, descended upon Washington demand-ing early payment. Unmoved by the "Bonus Army," as the marchers called themselves, Hoover dispatched regular Army troops led by General Douglas MacArthur to rout the ragtag brigade with tanks, bayonets, and tear gas.[3,4] The election wasn't close. Franklin carried forty-two states, winning 472 elec-toral votes to Hoover's 59.

Franklin was now in need of a presidential physician and asked his old friend Cary Grayson for help in finding one. Medical competence and the ability to keep a secret were top priorities. Grayson chose Ross T. McIntire, a 43-year-old career Navy medical officer with an impressive curriculum vitae.

A native of Salem, Oregon, McIntire received his medical degree in 1912 from that city's Willamette University. He had spent five years in private prac-tice when America entered World War I, whereupon he enlisted in the Navy Medical Corps as a lieutenant junior grade. McIntire met Grayson during the war and was impressed by the senior officer's empathy and demeanor. The younger man served aboard the cruiser USS *New Orleans*, which after the armistice became the U.S. station ship at Vladivostok, Russia. After a stint at a naval hospital in the Philippines, McIntire returned stateside in 1920 for postgraduate training in ophthalmology and otolaryngology, then was assigned to run the eye, ear, nose, and throat department at the naval hospital in San Diego.[5] He returned to sea duty in 1924 aboard USS *Relief*, the first pur-pose-built American hospital ship, which served the Pacific fleet. The next year he was transferred to the U.S. Naval Dispensary in Washington, D.C., under Grayson's command, where the two men developed a close relationship. "A kinder, more thoughtful man I never knew," McIntire later recalled. "Grayson came to me with poor devils in need of an operation, begging to know if I could do the necessary surgery outside and away from my regular duties. And always the hospital bills came out of his private purse."[6] After another tour at sea, in 1931 McIntire, now a lieutenant commander, was assigned to the U.S.

---

3 Other members of MacArthur's force included George S. Patton and Dwight D. Eisenhow-er.

4 As president, Franklin opposed the bonus.

5 Eye, Ear, Nose, and Throat were then combined under one specialty. The formal split did not occur until 1979. McIntire is almost universally identified as an ENT specialist. It is important to remember that he was also trained in surgery of the eye.

6 McIntire, 55–56.

Naval Hospital in Washington, D.C., with additional duties as an instructor of ophthalmology and otolaryngology at the Naval Medical School.

"As one of Franklin Roosevelt's oldest and dearest friends, Grayson became an intimate after the 1932 election, and thought of me when the President asked him about a physician."[7] McIntire recalled in his 1946 memoir. But then he claimed that Grayson told him, "The President is as strong as a horse with the exception of a chronic sinus condition that makes him susceptible to colds. That's where you come in."[8] The knowledge that Franklin was treated for cancer as early as 1930 puts the lie to that story. Just as Dr. Heiter had been recruited three years earlier, Ross McIntire's expertise as a top notch eye, nose, and sinus surgeon made him the best man for the job.

Equally important, McIntire made no bones about what was expected of him as White House physician. "The health of the chief executive … is his own private business," he wrote, "These men are officers as well as physicians, and being subject to the iron discipline of the armed services, they can be counted on to keep a closed mouth about what they see and hear."[9]

Franklin added another title to McIntire's résumé in 1938—Surgeon General of the Navy and head of the Navy's Bureau of Medicine and Surgery—which included supervision of a band of top notch physicians and cutting-edge technical expertise. The assignment came with a promotion to rear admiral, jumping McIntire ahead of six higher-ranking officers.[10] It is probably not coincidental that the promotion came only after Grayson's death in 1938 from lymphoma.[11] Among the letters of condolence to Grayson's widow was one addressed to "Dear little Gertrude of long ago," from Mrs. Winthrop Rutherfurd, the former Lucy Mercer, who had befriended the Graysons during her cruises with Franklin aboard the presidential yacht *Sylph* twenty years earlier.[12]

---

7 *Ibid.*

8 *Ibid.*, 57.

9 *Ibid.*, 58.

10 *Associated Press*, November 28, 1938.

11 Grayson also used Bernard Baruch's South Carolina estate, Hobcaw Barony, to build strength prior to surgery for the cancer at the Mayo Clinic. Cary Grayson papers, Staunton, Virginia.

12 Cary Grayson papers, Woodrow Wilson birthplace, Staunton, Virginia.

■ Chapter 11
■ President-Elect

In February 1933, a month before Franklin's inauguration, the need for an operation performed under impenetrable secrecy brought Franklin aboard *Nourmahal* for the first time. He was surely aware of an unusual precedent. In July 1893, doctors had found a malignant tumor in President Grover Cleveland's upper jaw. A team of surgeons secretly and successfully excised the cancer aboard a private yacht, *Oneida*, owned by a wealthy friend of the President,[1] while the vessel was sailing on Long Island Sound. The surgeries, which included installation of a hard rubber prosthesis, remained hidden until eleven years after Cleveland's death when one of the doctors "W.W." Keen, told all in the *Saturday Evening Post* in September 1917.[2,3] Keen later misdiagnosed Franklin's polio at Campobello in 1921.

History repeated itself when Vincent Astor provided the venue for another secret surgery. The trip was billed as a restorative fishing vacation prior to Franklin's assumption of the presidency. On December 20, 1932, Vincent wrote to Dr. Heiter, "For obvious reasons, on this particular trip, it will be absolutely essential to have a member of your particular profession on board, and I don't know of anybody who would fit in as well as you." A revealing handwritten postscript added, "Our preliminary trip will have to be kept 'under the hat' until our principal guest gives it out."[4]

Nourmahal left Jacksonville, Florida, on February 4, 1933, sailed to the Bahamas, and returned on schedule to Miami on February 15. "In addition to the President [elect], on board were ['Nourmahal gang' members] Judge Frederic Kernochan, TR's son Kermit Roosevelt, George St. George [the husband of Franklin's cousin], William Rhinelander Stewart, Jr. [financier and renowned playboy],

---

1 Commodore Elias Cornelius Benedict was a prominent New York City banker and yachtsman.

2 Keen, W.W., "The Surgical Operations on President Cleveland." *Saturday Evening Post*, September 22, 1917. Keen's subsequent book included an apology to the reporter whose career had been negatively impacted for simply publishing a truthful story about the operation.

3 For a detailed history of the event, see: https://magicmastsandsturdyships.weebly.com/president-grover-clevelandx27s-secret-surgery-on-the-steam-yacht-oneida.html.

4 Heiter papers.

and Dr. Leslie Heiter ... Dr. Heiter, a great friend of mine, acted more or less as the ship's medical officer,"[5] Astor wrote to Grace Tully in 1949.[6] Also signing the ship's log were Secret Service agents Gus Gennerich, Bob Clark, and James Reidy, as well as Franklin's African-American valet, Irwin McDuffie, who had replaced Leroy Jones in 1927.[7] "At the very bottom of the list is a footprint of a dog which the President insisted on inserting," Astor wrote. "It represents my dachshund, Robin, whose foot the President pressed against an ink pad and then made a print in the [log]."

"On the evening of our return to Miami the President addressed a large open-air meeting of the American Legion," Astor wrote. "And it was on this occasion that a lunatic [bricklayer Giuseppe Zangara] fired, as I remember, five shots at him that fortunately missed but fatally wounded Mayor Czermak [sic] of Chicago who was standing about two feet from the President." The *Nourmahal* party had left the dock in a five-car caravan for Miami's Bayfront Park, where Franklin spoke from the back seat of an open car. Vincent went on to describe Franklin's bravery during the assassination attempt and his trip to the hospital while cradling the mortally wounded Cermak in his arms.

Another firsthand account of the event comes from Dr. Heiter, who wrote to his father the next day:

> "Dear Dad,
>
> Well you wanted a story and believe you me we gave it to the world last night. It was the most exciting night I've had in many a day if not ever. Arriving [in Miami] about dark, we were met by crowds lining the causeway all the way in, motor launches, planes, blimps and what have you. Then we settled down to a very quiet supper, the last of the [*Nourmahal*] party. Then off at 8:30 to hear the Governor make a speech—our car was the last in line of police escort, George St. George, the genial Judge [Kernochan] & I—well they stopped us at the park as you couldn't get near the place. So we decided to idle in the car out of hearing distance. Then all of a sudden, five sharp cracks & we noticed the crowd is beginning to mill & surge, someone shouting "Someone's shot"—So off I dash with George & Freddy [Kernochan] at my heels, to be stopped point blank by the Shriners who were keeping everyone out. No manner of argument could convince them that I was the Doc, etc.—So we retreated having word that the

5 Vincent Astor to Grace Tully, 1949, Tully papers, FDRL.
6 Grace Tully papers, FDRL.
7 https://www.whitehousehistory.org/presidential-valets.

Pres-elect had been taken off in another car. Up to the county jail goes I to see what hospital the wounded had been taken to[8]—and while there waiting telephone communication in they dump the would be assassin kerplunk! on the floor [inside a burlap sack][9]—by that time I have the word and off we go again across town to the hospital—so 50 miles per h. thru traffic arriving there to find Vincent pacing up & down the corridor—calling me—The Mayor took me in and was I glad to see Vincent okay, for up to that time I didn't know who had been shot—then he said the Gov was Okay but that Pres-elect wanted me to offer my services to Cermak—which we did but they didn't relish it much. Naturally the town Doctors had taken him over and they were going ahead with x-raying which was about all that could be done at that time anyhow. So I just stuck around, looked at the pictures etc.—Then Mrs. Gill [a bystander Zangara had shot in the abdomen] was operated on at once—she's quite desperate today, has had two transfusions. Cermak's bullet went thru the rib and is lodged in one of his vertebrae, unless something unforeseen occurs I believe he will make it okay.[10] The rest of them are doing very well—We went up this morning—The Pres. Vincent and I—thru streets with 500 Secret Service men on all sides—cops everywhere. It was quite a kick. Then we paraded back downtown to the station—and was the Gov. tired when we reached the station. We were all pretty well done in last night. We didn't get to bed until about 2:30 for after coming from the hospital, I had to draw pictures & explain what was going on to the Gov. [FDR] until the wee hour of 2 a.m. & was plenty tired."

"He's gone now—left at 10 this a.m. and what a job he is taking over—Whew! I wouldn't be in his place for plenty of money. He showed his stuff under fire the last night—I'm all for him. When we parted this a.m. he said 'Les, make Vincent take Asst. Sect. of the Navy & do what you can.' (Quiet on that) We're off tomorrow for Havana—one day there I think and to Panama—Love Les"[11]

Vincent later gave a flawed account of the assassination attempt to free-lance writer Sidney Shalett, who was collaborating with Franklin's son

---

8 Police headquarters was located on the nineteenth floor of Miami's City Hall. Davis, K.S. *FDR the New York Years 1928-1933.* New York: Random House, 1959, 431.

9 The would-be assassin was Giuseppe Zangara, an unemployed bricklayer. Zangara was subsequently interviewed in his jail cell by Judge Frederic Kernochan.

10 Cermak's wounds were initially not felt to be fatal as the bullet had lodged harmlessly in one of his vertebra. Unfortunately, though, it had also lacerated a bowel and Cermak died of peritonitis from the leak nineteen days later.

11 Heiter papers.

James on his memoir, *Affectionately FDR*.[12] On December 3, 1958, James had written to Dr. Heiter to fact-check his draft manuscript, seeking to confirm Vincent's version of the story "in the interest of complete accuracy."[13] Astor had been under the incorrect assumption that a policeman had arrested Heiter, suspecting him of being a co-conspirator—and locked him in a cell with Zangara *"because no one would believe you that you were the President's doctor"* (emphasis added). "That's not the way it happened, but Vincent liked to tell it that way," said Heiter's son Bill, curator of his father's papers.[14] As published, *Affectionately FDR* describes the members of the *Nourmahal* gang with thumbnail biographies. Dr. Heiter has been intentionally eliminated—with the exception of his name in a photo caption.

A high-resolution photograph of Franklin sitting with Hoover in the back seat of their open car on Inauguration Day, March 4, 1933, reveals a distinct linear scar within Franklin's left lateral eyebrow below the base of the triangular pigmented lesion first seen in 1923—evidence of a surgical procedure likely performed by Dr. Heiter aboard *Nourmahal* less than a month earlier. Franklin's eyebrow would later serve as an easily camouflaged portal for multiple surgeries performed by Ross McIntire.[15]

---

12 The book was released on January 1, 1959. Vincent died on February 3, 1959 at age 67.

13 James Roosevelt to Les Heiter, December 3, 1958. Heiter papers.

14 Author's interview with Bill Heiter, 2018.

15 A twenty-seven-minute video exquisitely documenting the growth and staged surgical removal of the melanoma is posted online at https://www.youtube.com/watch?v=udM4bPU5q2Q.

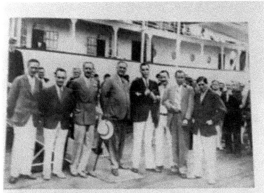

The "Nourmahal Gang," 1933. Left to right: Lytle Hull, Dr. Leslie Heiter, William Rhinelander Stewart, Father, Vincent Astor (owner of the yacht), Kermit Roosevelt, George St. George, and Justice Frederic Kernochan

FDR's first cruise aboard Nourmahal showing the "Nourmahal Gang" February 1933. Dr. Heiter seen at left.

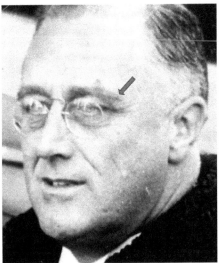

FDR at his first inauguration likely showing surgical scar created by Dr. Heiter a month earlier aboard the ship.

■ Chapter 12
■ Fear Itself

The weather in Washington, D.C. on the morning of March 4, 1933, was frigid and gloomy, matching the country's mood. Americans faced a future certain only in its bleakness. Bank failures and foreclosures on farms and homes were on the rise. The New York Stock Exchange and the Chicago Board of Trade had had to suspend trading.

The president-elect began his day attending a service conducted by his Groton headmaster, Rev. Endicott Peabody, at St. John's Episcopal Church, across Lafayette Square from the White House.[1] Franklin and Eleanor arrived at the White House at 11 a.m. in an open touring car to meet a dour Herbert Hoover, who acquiesced to tradition and rode with his successor on the one-and-a-half mile parade route to the Capitol. Franklin waved his silk top hat and flashed his famous grin in response to the cheering crowds. Hoover made little effort at collegiality. Another open car carrying their wives followed.[2]Insert Photo 12.1 Here

To camouflage Franklin's inability to walk, inaugural chairman Dr. Cary Grayson had had a wooden passageway constructed from the Capitol rotunda to the site of the swearing-in on the east front. Film of Franklin traversing the final thirty-five feet down a ramp to the speaker's podium shows his upper body swaying back and forth as he propelled himself down a ramp toward the lectern with James on his left, father and son using a variant of the technique they had developed in 1924 (by now, Franklin was strong enough to replace the crutch with a cane). Neither Franklin's cane nor his vice-like grip on James's arm is visible.

Even the oath of office had to be staged to create the impression Franklin was standing unassisted opposite Chief Justice Charles Evans Hughes—his right hand raised, his left surreptitiously grasping support, with the

---

1 Alter, 212–213.
2 This cover never ran. It was pulled at the last minute after Cermak died of the wound from Giuseppe Zangara's assassination attempt in Miami a month earlier. See: https://www.newyorker.com/news/amy-davidson/the-f-d-r-new-yorker-cover-that-never-ran (last accessed April 10, 2022).

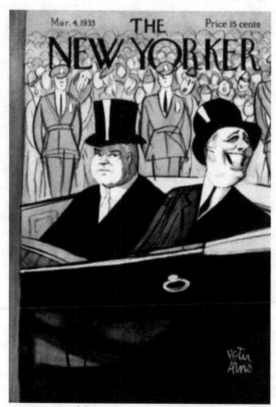

Anticipated but never used painting by Peter Arno for March 4, 1933 cover of The New Yorker.

seventeenth-century Dutch family Bible held open to the first epistle to the Corinthians before him.[3] Once he had been sworn in, the thirty-second president pivoted to grasp the specially constructed lectern with both hands and spoke the words which would become the most memorable he ever uttered: "This great nation will endure as it has endured, will revive, and will prosper ... let me assert my firm belief that the only thing we have to fear is—fear itself—nameless, unreasoning, unjustified terror which paralyzes needed efforts to convert retreat into advance," he said.[4]

Listening to their new president's patrician voice, people across the nation doubtless were thinking, "What does *he* know about fear?" He had never had to worry about going without a meal, losing a job, or being forced to abandon his home or farm. But Franklin *had* known fear. Illness had more than once brought him to the brink of death. Polio had left him unable to move normally—every time he went out in public he faced the prospect of falling flat on his face—and in 1930 he had heard the three most frightening words in the English language—You have cancer.[5] As Franklin was leaving the podium on James's arm, a sunbeam broke through the clouds. A witness wrote in his diary, "it came to rest, like a friendly hand, upon his head."

---

3 Franklin was the first president to repeat the Chief Justices words aloud.
4 "Fear itself" was not as impactful a statement as it might have seemed. It took some time for the phrase to reach its iconic status.
5 FDR was by no means the first in his family to have cancer. His maternal grandmother, Catherine Lyman Delano, died of lung cancer at 71 as did Eleanor's paternal grandfather who succumbed to a gastric malignancy at age 46, not revealing his diagnosis to his son Theodore, the future President, until the latest stages of the disease.

Chapter 13
Building a New Deal

Missy LeHand, Franklin's de facto chief of staff, and Louis Howe put together the new administration's infrastructure in five months—which included Missy's recommendation for a new Attorney General after the original nominee, Montana Senator Thomas Walsh, died of a heart attack en route to the inauguration after a honeymoon with his younger bride.[1] Missy occupied the office adjacent to Franklin's in the White House and controlled virtually all access to him.

Congress was ready to act. The Senate confirmed the cabinet without hearings. For the first time, that body included a woman—Secretary of Labor Frances Perkins. "Roosevelt assumed leadership during one of the greatest crises in modern history—a crisis that seemed to mark the total breakdown of the American system—and his response to that emergency changed the nation's ways forever," *Time* magazine wrote at the centennial of Franklin's birth. "In the tumultuous period still known as the Hundred Days, he pushed a broad array of legislation through Congress, ranging from reform of the nation's banks to the reorganization of the entire farm system."

Americans terrified of bank failures were emptying their savings accounts. Franklin brainstormed with Secretary of the Treasury William Woodin, Attorney General Homer Cummings, and top economic adviser Raymond Moley to plan a dramatic move—a "bank holiday." Institutional financial activities would be shut down for four days.

During the mandatory intermezzo, which began on March 9, Congress passed the Emergency Banking Act. This first piece of New Deal legislation authorized the Federal Reserve to issue additional currency to cover any further withdrawals and provided a federal guarantee of 100 percent of the money held in depositors' accounts. The law also applied new rules to the stock market, created jobs with government projects, and established loan programs for financially strapped farmers and homeowners.

---

1 Jonathan Daniels later said that Walsh died of "presumption beyond his powers." Smith, K., 123.

The night before the bank holiday was to end, sixty million people tuned in to Franklin's first "Fireside Chat" and heard his calm and reassuring voice. "I want to tell you what has been done in the last few days, why it was done and what the next steps are going to be," he said. "It is safer to keep your money in a reopened bank than it is under the mattress."[2] Americans listened. When banks reopened, customers began to redeposit the funds they had withdrawn.

Stephen T. Early, an original member of the Cuff Links Club, signed on as press secretary and assumed Louis Howe's role as chief spin-doctor, which included his highly underappreciated part in covering-up Franklin's health problems.[3] Early invented a new method of dealing with the media—the live, interactive presidential press conference.[4] The first of 998 such events took place on March 8.

Franklin was now the most photographed person in America. Efforts to erase the visual record of his disability were ramped up. His metal braces disappeared from newspaper and magazine photographs—painted black and concealed with extra-long trousers. At state dinners and speeches to Congress the president was seated before other guests arrived. The pretense was enhanced by a flood of commercially produced shelf clocks and lamps portraying him as "Man of the Hour," standing straight-legged behind a ship's wheel—steering the country forward.

Within months, farmers were bringing crops to market instead of burning them, factories were reopening, and relief programs were putting money into Americans' pockets. *The New York Times* Weekly Business Index, which had been 52.3 in March, reached 87.1 in mid-June. By no means was the Depression over, but for the first time in years there was at least some hope for the future. Not all New Deal initiatives succeeded but an American

---

2 Miller, 312.

3 Early was a key figure in the cover-up of Franklin's numerous health problems, especially during the protracted periods of absence for reasons of health in 1940 and 1941. The scrapbook he kept is a valuable source of untapped information and contains rarely cited transcripts of his own interactions with reporters. A descendant of Confederate General Jubal Early, with "Pa" Watson Early was one of the southern contingent of FDR's inner circle. He was likely responsible for introducing FDR to urologist William Calhoun Stirling. A 2008 biography by Linda Lotridge Levin *The Making of FDR: The Story of Stephen T. Early, America's First Modern Press Secretary*, does not touch on his important role in the cover-up.

4 Herbert Hoover had answered written questions submitted by reporters, but FDR was the first to take them face to face.

public desperate for action was happy to see them in any form. If (Roosevelt) burned down the Capitol we would cheer and say, "Well, we at least got a fire started anyhow," humorist Will Rogers quipped.[5]

No one was better at putting people to work than Harry Hopkins. Franklin brought him to Washington as federal relief administrator. Convinced that paid work was psychologically more valuable than cash handouts, Hopkins used the blueprint of New York's TERA program to create FERA, the Federal Emergency Relief Administration, which dispensed money across the nation for work relief projects. Hopkins also supervised the Civil Works Administration (CWA), which hired four million people during its five months of operation. CWA's successor, the extraordinarily successful Works Progress Administration (WPA), put 8.5 million people to work during its seven-year history—constructing schools, hospitals, airports, parks, playgrounds, bridges, dams, public buildings, stadiums, golf courses, and over 650,000 miles of highways and roads. Hopkins also created the National Youth Administration to assist teenagers, and "Federal One" programs for artists, writers, musicians, and actors. One of the earliest and most popular New Deal initiatives, the Civilian Conservation Corps (CCC), would eventually provide food, housing, and medical care for three million young men working in forestry, prevention of soil erosion, and flood control, as well as the construction of hundreds of state parks and upgrades of national parks.

In 1933, Franklin's Brain Trust added a new group of Harvard law professors recruited by their colleague Felix Frankfurter. Among them were the "Gold Dust Twins," policy wonk Benjamin V. Cohen, and his associate Thomas P. Corcoran, a gregarious political savant who replaced an ailing Louis Howe as Franklin's "fixer" and became one of his most influential political advisers.[6]

The 1934 mid-term elections solidified the Democrats' hold on Congress. Frances Perkins was appointed to lead a commission assigned to recommend how to ensure the economic welfare of all Americans. A program of "social security" was proposed to provide benefits for retirees and their survivors, as well as insurance for the unemployed and the disabled—a policy particularly close to Franklin's heart. Social Security was self-funded through an income tax to obviate criticism of the program as being socialist.

---

5 Schlessinger, A., *The Coming of the New Deal, 1933–1935*. New York: Houghton Mifflin, 1958, 13.
6 McKean, D., *Peddling Influence. Thomas "Tommy the Cork" Corcoran and the Birth of Modern Lobbying.* Hanover, NH: Steerforth Press, 2005.

Hopkins's successes brought him into Franklin's inner circle. He was being groomed as a possible running mate until doctors diagnosed him with advanced cancer of the stomach. Surgery at the Mayo Clinic in December 1937[7,8] miraculously cured his malignancy—which even today kills 70 percent of its victims within five years.[9] Hopkins recovered well enough to be named Secretary of Commerce in 1938 but severe inability to take in nutrition continued to plague him. In 1939, the Mayo Clinic sent him home to die, whereupon "Old Dr. Roosevelt" turned his friend "Harry the Hop"[10] over to the doctors at Ross McIntire's Naval Bureau of Medicine and Surgery. A team led by tropical disease specialist and former Navy Surgeon General Rear Admiral Edward R. Stitt kept Hopkins alive and productive until his death in 1946.[11]

7 Halsted, J.A., "Severe Malnutrition in a Public Servant of the World War II Era: The Medical History of Harry Hopkins." Transactions of the American Clinical and Climatological Association 1975;86:23–32. Halsted was Anna Roosevelt's third husband.

8 Pappas, T.N., Swanson, S., "The Life, Times, and Health Care of Harry L Hopkins: Presidential Advisor and Perpetual Patient." Journal of Medical Biography 2018;26(1): 49–59.

9 https://www.cancer.org/cancer/stomach-cancer/detection-diagnosis-staging/survival-rates.html.

10 Franklin' affectionately devised nicknames for a number of his most important circle of advisers. Tom Corcoran became "Tommy the Cork"; Harry Hopkins "Harry the Hop"; Henry Morganthau "Henry the Morgue"; Harold Ickes "Donald Duck." Marrin, A., FDR and the American Crisis. South Bend, IN: Ember, 2016, 126.

11 McIntire's Bureau literally invented new ways of putting weight on Hopkins. He underwent over fifty transfusions, most at the White House, where he was living between 1940 and 1943. Hopkins eventually died from complications of the transfusions—cirrhosis of the liver due to viral hepatitis—a disease not discovered until long after his death. Yet another interesting medical twist is described here for the first time: Anna Roosevelt Halsted died in 1975 of mouth cancer. Her husband at the time was James Halsted. After her death, Halsted married Hopkin's daughter, Joyce, who also developed oral cancer. This raises the probability that Halsted infected both of his wives with Human Papilloma Virus (HPV), now known to be associated with the disease. Pytynia, K.B., Dahlstrom, R., Sturgis, E.M., "Epidemiology of HPV-Associated Oropharyngeal Cancer." Oral Oncology May 2014;50(5):380–386.

■ Chapter 14

■ "Our Little Alabama Doctor"

On August 3, 1933, a friendly letter from Vincent Astor to Franklin made reference to Dr. Heiter as "our little Alabama doctor."[1] On August 31, Franklin joined Astor, Heiter, and five other members of the *Nourmahal* Gang at Poughkeepsie, New York, for Franklin's second voyage aboard the yacht—a six-day cruise on the Gulf Stream. Little is known of events on this voyage other than "extraordinarily poor fishing."[2] After the trip, Franklin treated his sailing companions to dinner and a movie at the White House.[3]

The primary purpose of Franklin's third *Nourmahal* cruise was to treat his melanoma with radiation. The president had to be sequestered to recover from a secret medical procedure. The yacht was scheduled to depart Jacksonville for the Bahamas on March 28, 1934.[4] Uncharacteristically, Franklin's oldest son, James, would be on board. The trip was ostensibly a nine-day fishing vacation which included an Easter service Franklin planned to conduct aboard ship— the first president to do so. *Nourmahal* was supposed to dock at Miami on the morning of Friday April 6, when Franklin would board a train to Washington. On April 7, he was to meet with the President of Haiti and that evening be guest of honor at the Gridiron Club dinner, a high-profile annual event sponsored by The Washington Press Club.

On March 27, a telegram addressed to "President Roosevelt" arrived at the White House from Dr. H. B. McEuen, director of a cancer radiotherapy treatment center at Jacksonville's St. Luke's Hospital.[5] McEuen had invented a portable machine to deliver high-voltage x-irradiation.[6] The telegram requested a meeting "relative to treatment of the cancer patient"[7] aboard *Nourmahal* just

---

1 Astor to FDR, August 3, 1933 Grace Tully papers. FDRL, Box 116.
2 Astor to Grace Tully. June 28, 1949. Grace Tully Papers, FDRL.
   Trips of the President, FDRL.
3 FDR, Day by Day, September 5, 1933.
4 Trips of the President, FDRL.
5 The Astor family had been benefactors of the facility for three generations.
6 The device still exists, confirmed in a telephone conversation between the author and H.B. "Tripp" McEuen III.
7 Trips of the President, FDRL.

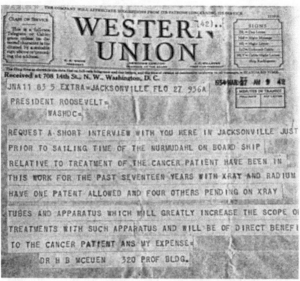

February 17, 1934 telegram from Dr. H.B. McEuen to FDR touting his portable radiation machine as being of great benefit to the cancer patient.

before the yacht sailed to demonstrate how the device worked, claiming his apparatus "will be of direct benefit to the cancer patient [repetition in text]."[8]

In 1930, McEuen had published a "Report of Six Cases of Malignant Melanoma Treated with X-radiation, with Two Cases Cured for Over Five Years" in America's leading radiological journal.[9] The article likely caught the attention of Dr. Heiter, who had trained at Memorial Hospital under Dr. James Ewing, America's foremost cancer doctor, who was a strong advocate of treating the disease with radiation.

Escort for the cruise was to be provided by destroyer USS *Ellis*, with additional support from a navy seaplane based in Miami. A triangular net of radio communications was established between Washington, *Ellis*, and another destroyer, USS *Tattnall*, which was to be anchored at Miami near the Biltmore Hotel, where Marvin McIntyre had set up press headquarters. There was also

---

8 Trips of the President, FDRL.
9 McEuen, H.B., "Report of Six Cases of Malignant Melanoma Treated with X-Radiation, with Two Cases Cured for Over Five Years." *Radiology* June 1, 1930;14:6.

an open telegraph line established between McIntyre and the White House. "The president is within a few minutes contact at all times with Washington," the Associated Press reported.[10]

Dr. Heiter likely used Dr. McEuen's machine on March 28. "Had fine night," *Nourmahal* reported the next morning, "The president expects to spend the day fishing and having a swim."[11] At 7:30 p.m. on March 29, a coded message indicated the patient was doing well. "Now under way for Nassau after good fishing day," Vincent wired McIntyre.

At 9 a.m. Friday, March 30, *Nourmahal* arrived at Nassau, Bahamas, to a 21-gun salute from British cruiser HMS *Danae*.[12,13] Governor Sir Bede Clifford, accompanied by his wife and daughter, called on Franklin aboard ship. James departed *Nourmahal* for Palm Beach, Florida aboard the Navy seaplane.[14] At a party given in his honor the next day by Joseph P. Kennedy, James informed reporters his father was having a "fine fishing trip."[15]

On Easter Sunday morning, April 1, *Nourmahal* anchored off San Salvador Island,[16] where Franklin welcomed the officers and crew of *Ellis* for a divine service. The subject of his homily was the divine guidance God had given Christopher Columbus to discover the New World. Franklin

---

10 "Close communication is being maintained with Washington. And open telegraph wires established in the Miami Biltmore hotel connected with the White House. Radio connections are maintained both through the *Nourmahal* and the destroyer Ellis and the president is within a few minutes contact at all times with Washington." ((AP) *The Plain Speaker*, Hazleton Pa., April 3, 1934); During the Easter Service, "a wire connecting the White House was open here with the veteran Ed Smithers of the White House staff, on this end of the line. Mr. Roosevelt is in very close contact with the capital" (*Miami News*, April 2, 1934).
11 *Associated Press*, March 29, 1934.
12 *Associated Press*, April 1, 1934.
13 Guns Boom in Salute as FDR Enters Tropics. *United Press*, March 31, 1934.
14 *Ibid.*
15 "James Roosevelt Says Dad is Having Fine Fishing Trip." *Palm Beach Post*, April 1, 1934.
16 Known as Watling's Island from the 1680s until 1925.

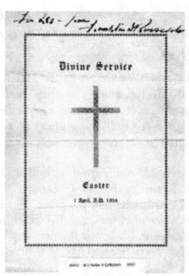

Cover of program FDR's Easter 1934 divine service aboard Nuormahal inscribed to Dr. Heiter.

inscribed a copy of the program "For Les," his physician and friend, Dr. Heiter.[17,18,19]

The earliest indication of a serious problem on *Nourmahal* came late in the afternoon of Monday, April 2, when Steve Early announced in Washington that the Gridiron Club dinner had been postponed. Most likely, Franklin's radiation treatment had unexpectedly caused a hemorrhage into one of his sinuses.[20] At 8:26 p.m. McIntyre relayed a message sent by Franklin to Early,

---

17 Heiter collection.

18 *New York Daily News* columnist John O'Donnell provided a description. "For the first time in history the President of the United States acting in his capacity as commander-in-chief of the navy, conducted church services this Easter Sunday morning on the quarter deck of the pleasure craft. Officers and men of the destroyer *Ellis*, convoying the presidential craft, boarded the *Nourmahal* and lined up on the afterdeck with Vincent Astor, the crew of 30 officers and men of the *Nourmahal* and the guests invited by Astor to join the fishing expedition. When the congregation was assembled, the chaplain's flag was run up above the national ensign and Mr. Roosevelt read the services from the book of common prayer." "Notes from the Florida White House." *Salt Lake Tribune*, April 1, 1934.

19 Heiter Collection.

20 The news got to Washington directly from *Nourmahal/Ellis*. No transcript of the message

"Please phone White House and get list of my appointments and dinners next week. Could President Haiti be postponed until latter part of week?"

The cover-up began late on April 2. Early informed the press, "Mr. Roosevelt is thoroughly enjoying himself and wishes to take advantage of his present vacation period to store up the energy needed for the long grind before Congress adjourned in May or June."[21]

After news of the Gridiron postponement reached Miami, McIntyre telegraphed Early at 9:23 p.m.: "Boys all getting queries rumors Boss sick etc, resulting speculation about postponement Gridiron dinner. I've sent several messages to the Boss keeping him posted and asking for decision about return trip. So far no replies. Guess only thing to do wait hear from him. Elliott here, going out tomorrow to boat. Geo. Hearst with him but not going out.[22] Don't suppose you know anything more than I do."

Thirty minutes later, Early sent the official excuse to McIntyre. "Gridiron Club postponed dinner to Saturday, April fourteenth. Have assured them president will attend that date. Club postponed dinner hoping extension of time would enable president complete vacation and secure needed and deserved rest before returning here to continue his strenuous labor. Please advise the President."

In consequence, McIntyre sent *Nourmahal* an urgent, confidential, coded radio message: "Newspaper men being queried of home office on announcement one week postponement of Gridiron dinner. They wish to know if this

---

has surfaced.

21 *New York Times*, April 2, 1934.
22 Elliott had been en route to Miami since March 30 from Los Angeles, first by train to Fort Worth to drop off his eight-months pregnant wife at her mother's home on April 1, then joined by plane there by his boss George Hearst who had flown in from Los Angeles on a commercial Ford Trimotor. After meeting up in Fort Worth on Easter Sunday, the two famous children had reached Shreveport, Louisiana by 6 p.m. aboard a private Bellanca CH 400 "Skyrocket" piloted by aviation pioneer Theodore Nieman "Ted" Kincanon. The trio began the final 1,100-mile leg to Miami at 6 a.m. Tuesday April 2, stopped to refuel in Alabama, and reached Miami by late evening. Kincanon (b. August 16, 1896) died in a plane crash in a snowstorm near Dallas on January 29, 1936 but his five passengers survived. On April 12, 1937 he was posthumously awarded the Airmail Flyers Medal of Honor by President Roosevelt. See: https://en.wikipedia.org/wiki/Theodore_%22Ted%22_ Nieman_Kincannon. Exactly why Elliot and Hearst made the trip from Los Angeles to Miami is unclear. The two men went on to Washington shortly after Elliott's return from meeting his father.

means extension of your trip. Steve, Louis and I feel [it is] vitally important you stay until middle or latter part of the week. Please advise."

FDR's son Elliott had showed up in Miami on April 2 with George Hearst, the son of media magnate William Randolph Hearst. The next day, Tuesday, April 3, at 11:41 a.m., Astor sent a coded dispatch to McIntyre: "Arrived all well off Elbow Key after a fine night at sea. The President is awaiting the arrival of Jimmy and Elliott and later we all hope to give the fish [FDR] an active afternoon."[23],[24] "Active afternoon" likely refers to a blood transfusion.[25]

"Mr. Astor's general report that all was well aboard the *Nourmahal* received credence in the opinion of officials and observers here from the fact that the *Nourmahal* is still at sea," *The New York Times* reported from Miami on April 3. "Had the President shown the least symptom of illness, it was thought by his aides here that the *Nourmahal* would have rushed to port or likely had brought about medical aid from shore."[26] Unbeknownst to the press, Dr. Heiter had been administering that "medical aid," most probably cauterizing blood vessels and packing Franklin's nose with iodine-infused gauze to control the hemorrhage.[27]

At 2:45 p.m. on April 3, Early wired Vincent that reaction to news of the prolonged vacation was "generally excellent," and suggested Franklin personally thank Gridiron Club president, James L. Wright, for making it possible to extend his cruise. "Wright Message should be phrased that it can be published and will convince the few who profess to see illness as cause of delayed return." Early and McIntyre later decided the thank you note was not necessary. At 4 p.m. Franklin's sons Elliott and James arrived at Elbow Key after a 160-mile seaplane flight from Miami.[28]

Elliott stayed at the anchorage for little more than an hour, probably to give blood, then returned to Miami to spin a fairy tale to reporters about his father's

23 Trips of the President, FDRL.
24 *Ibid.*
25 For a detailed discussion of Astor's fascination with espionage and codes, see Persico, J., *Roosevelt's Secret War: FDR and World War II Espionage*. New York: Random House, 2001, 9–13.
26 *New York Times*, April 3, 1934.
27 A debt of thanks is owed to Robert Ruben, MD, Professor and Chairman emeritus of ENT at NYC's Montefiore Medical Center, for his help about how sinus hemorrhage would have been treated in 1934.
28 *Bergen Record*, April 6, 1934.

SONS VISIT PRESIDENT ON CRUISE

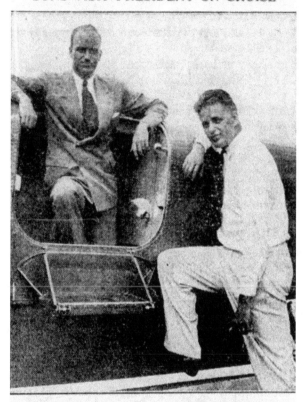

—Associated Press Phot

James (left) and Elliott Roosevelt, sons of President Roosevel ire shown as they boarded a navy plane at Miami, Fla., to fly ou o the yacht, Nourmahal, to visit their father who is enjoying a fish ng cruise in Southern waters. On his return Elliott reported h ather "feeling swell" but catching no fish. The President joshing! lemanded a retraction of the latter statement.

April 3, 1943 AP news photo of James and Elliott Roosevelt confirming their seaplane flight to Nourmahal.

poor fishing luck. Jimmy remained behind aboard *Nourmahal*. "Elliott just returned," McIntyre wired Early at 7:30 p.m. "He gave nice interview to the boys, also dispelling rumors of illness, injury, etc, also told me confidentially his father would send in a story about his plans for extending his vacation. Everything O.K."[29] At 8:42 p.m., Astor wired McIntyre from *Ellis*: "Jimmy and Elliott arrived all well at four this afternoon. All greatly enjoyed Sunday papers and our mail delivered by plane. Conditions here seem ideal so planning remain another day perhaps longer."[30] At 10:35 p.m. Astor added, "Thanks to you [McIntyre] Elliott fed all the gulf fish. In consequence huge success."[31]

Also on April 3, Dr. Heiter sent a carefully worded letter to his father to explain the delay in his return to Alabama: "Vincent tells me that perhaps the President will stay on until early next week, and if so it means I will have to also. Duty, etc., etc., but the man is tired and really needs to rest."[32]

Franklin was probably still bleeding the next day. Another coded message on Wednesday, April 4, read "Remaining on at present anchorage and in pursuit of elusive Marlin to duplicate last nite success." Dr. Heiter got the hemorrhage under control later that day. "Much improvement in situation since last message, Everyone happy," Vincent and Jimmy radioed Washington. Early relayed the message to McIntyre in an urgent, confidential telegram.[33]

He followed up with a phone call to McIntyre to fill in the details, then reminded his colleague to keep his mouth shut: "Last message refers to report I gave you over the phone. Saying nothing here and know you won't."[34]

"There were widespread reports throughout the country today, that the president had become ill," *The New York Times* reported, "but several hours after the original inquiries had been sent to the *Nourmahal* a vague negative reply was sent to Marvin H. McIntyre, assistant White House secretary, by Vincent Astor, owner of the *Nourmahal* who reported 'all well and happy' aboard the ship."

29 Trips of the President, FDRL.
30 *Ibid.*
31 *Ibid.*
32 Heiter Collection.
33 Trips of the President, FDRL.
34 *Ibid.*

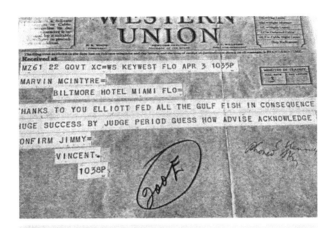

WESTERN UNION

Received at

MZ61 22 GOVT XC=WS KEYWEST FLO APR 3 1035P

MARVIN MCINTYRE=

BILTMORE HOTEL MIAMI FLO=

THANKS TO YOU ELLIOTT FED ALL THE GULF FISH IN CONSEQUENCE
HUGE SUCCESS BY JUDGE PERIOD GUESS HOW ADVISE ACKNOWLEDGE
CONFIRM JIMMY=

VINCENT-

1038P

TELEGRAM

The White House
Washington

HUSH   CONFIDENTIAL   April 4, 1934

TELEGRAPHIC MEMO TO McINTYRE

        Just received at five naught five pm the following message
signed Jimmy Vincent quote Much improvement in situation since last
message Everyone happy unquote

                                STEVE

TELEGRAM

The White House
Washington

                                    April 4, 1934

CONFIDENTIAL MEMO TO McINTYRE

        Last message refers to report I gave you over t?
phone stop Saying nothing here and know you wont.

                                STEVE

*Corrrespondence to and From Nourmahial April
1934 confirming the cover-up of FDR's acute illnes.*

97

Elliott's fishing ruse worked to perfection. *Time* magazine used the cruise as a setting for its April 9, 1934, feature story about Vincent's close relationship with Franklin. One passenger mentioned in the article was "Dr. Leslie Heiter of Mobile, Ala., a friend of Vincent Astor, present in a professional as well as a social capacity."

"Last week Franklin D. Roosevelt, finding that he needed more rest than even he had thought, decided to add a week to his fishing trip aboard Vincent Astor's *Nourmahal*," the article said.[35] There all last week he sat alert at the end of two long strings. One string, strong and tightly braided, slanted off into the pale green waters of the Gulf Stream. The other string, more tenuous and even longer, a string of radio messages and mail planes, soared off to distant Miami.

"To both strings he had to pay heed. A tug on one meant that a grouper or a marlin, coming up from the deep, was demanding the most careful attention of the President of the U. S. A tug on the other meant that something in Washington was also coming up to demand Rooseveltian attention. So content was the President in minding his strings that certain good citizens began to worry about the state of his health: rumors began to circulate of illness or injury to him.

"They were summarily disposed of when a Navy seaplane carrying a cockpitful of dispatches and two Roosevelt sons—Elliott who had flown from Texas in company with George Hearst and James who had been ashore for two days to visit Bostonian Joseph P. Kennedy—flew out to the *Nourmahal*, anchored off Elbow Cay. A few hours later Elliott flew back to Miami and told newshawks that:

1 His father was getting sunburned and had never been in better health or spirits.

2 His father's fishing luck was rotten. He had been fishing all morning with Secret Servant Robert Clark. Sleuth Clark had caught three barracuda, the President none.

"That evening President Roosevelt, sitting on the quarterdeck of the *Nourmahal* with his socialite fishing friends—Frederic Kernochan, George St. George, William Rhinelander Stewart, Lytle Hull, Cousin Kermit Roosevelt, host Vincent Astor [Dr. Heiter's name is now conspicuously absent.]—was chagrined to hear issuing from a radio the voice of

35 *Time*, April 16, 1934.

Newscaster Lowell Thomas telling the nation that the President of the U. S., on the authority of his own son, was fishing without success."

"Next day Host Astor dispatched an indignant radio message that shook Secretary Marvin McIntyre from pleasant relaxation and lethargy in Miami: "Heard Lowell Thomas relate Elliott's gross libel on President's fishing luck. He said appoint special committee to investigate and secure retraction." Later Host Astor pridefully dispatched another message: "Took 21 fish today."

"Secretary McIntyre, who between golf games was peacefully holding down the Miami end of the President's string of communications, went out grinning and gave the dispatches to the newshawks who for ten days had been sunning their hides without so much as one glimpse of the President. They snatched at the opportunity, radioed offering their services as a fish investigating committee—a gentle hint that it was about time the President gave them some news. The answer came back: 'Your generous unselfish suggestion received with pleasure … Fishing data on hand. Witnesses will waive immunity, Franklin D. Roosevelt.'"

To squelch any lingering doubts about Franklin's health, McIntyre brought reporters on a private boat to rendezvous with *Nourmahal* off Bimini Island on Friday, April 6. Franklin held court on the yacht's fantail, confining his comments to a lecture about local geography and an inventory of the party's catch. Despite the lighthearted performance, the official transcript of the event began: "The principal purpose of the visit of the press was to determine the state of health of the President. There had been rumors that he was very ill, et cetera, and they desired to disaffirm these rumors by eye-witness accounts."[36]

The caption of a photograph of the press conference reads: "President Roosevelt, on board the Astor yacht *Nourmahal*, joshingly denies for the benefit of reporters the statements of his son that he was not catching any fish on his vacation trip, and indicates the size of just one of the many he caught. He even went so far as to admit that he had caught a sperm whale with a three-ounce rod."[37]

---

36 Press Conferences of the President number 110, April 9, 1934, FDRL.

37 In full: President Roosevelt, on board the Astor yacht *Nourmahal*, joshingly denies for the benefit of reporters the statements of his son that he was not catching any fish on his vacation and indicates the size of just one of the many he caught. He even went so far as to admit that he had caught a sperm whale with a three-ounce rod.

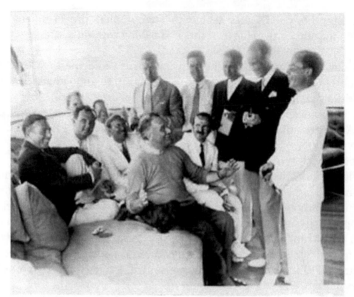

Press conference aboard Nourmahal, April 1934 given to promote "fish libel" deception.

McIntyre wrote to Kermit Roosevelt Jr. on April 11 to tell him that Joseph P. Kennedy, with whom Jimmy had been staying, would brief him on details of the event.[38] *"'Robbie' was really very, very ill* (emphasis added), as Joe will explain."[39,40] The press conference photo provides a clue to the identity of "Robbie," obviously an alias. Snuggled under Franklin's right elbow lays Astor's pet dachshund, Robin, AKA "Robbie," whose paw print Franklin had personally impressed in the official log of an earlier cruise.

---

38 Trips of the President, FDRL.

39 Kennedy made no mention of FDR's health in a contemporary memorandum. Merriman Smith, p. 127.

40 It is interesting to speculate whether Kennedy used his knowledge of Franklin's health to further his own agenda. Only two months later he was surprisingly named the first chairman of FDR's Security and Exchange Commission. Of Irish descent, his unlikely and ill-fated stint as Ambassador to the Court of St. James is well appreciated. JPK, with his Boston roots, may have also been the one who introduced FDR to Frank Lahey. One of the doctors who treated Missy LeHand in 1941 was psychiatrist James Watts, who later performed the disastrous pre-frontal lobotomy on JPK's daughter Rosemary.

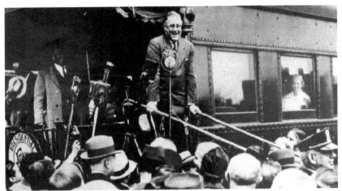

FDR arriving in Washington April 13, 1934 after his extended "vacation". Note Eleanor seen seated through train window.

Nourmahal docked at Miami on April 12. At the press conference aboard the train to Jacksonville, Franklin told reporters "I fished the first two days, caught a cold in my nose, slept a couple of days, then fishing and some more lazying around,"[41] He also mentioned "razzing the commodore" about his little dog.

Franklin arrived at Washington's Union Station on April 13, to a welcome by a festive crowd that included family, Louis Howe, disguised as a member of the band, and members of the cabinet and Congress.[42]

"I can't be truthful and say I am glad to get back," Franklin said. "I expected on this trip to get some good publicity about the fish I was catching ... I did have a wonderful holiday and I have come back with all sorts of new lessons which I've learned from barracudas and sharks. I am a tough guy!"[43]

There were no further questions as to why the President of the United States had extended a ten-day vacation to sixteen. Elliott never said anything further about "fish libel."[44] Jimmy, though, went to great lengths to keep his father's

---

41 Press Conferences of the President, Number 111, April 12, 1934, FDRL.

42 FDR Day by Day, April 13, 1934.

43 Dallek, R., *Franklin D. Roosevelt. A Political Life*. New York: Viking, 201. Taken from multiple sources including Burns and Schlesinger. A video is also available in the Pare Lorenz archive at the FDRL.

44 The nature of Elliott's "business trip" with George Hearst is unknown. He had left his home in Los Angeles by train for Dallas, before *Nourmahal* embarked, to bring his eight-month pregnant wife to her mother's home. Ruth Chandler Roosevelt was born in Fort

1934 medical episode secret. In a blatant attempt to rewrite history, his 1959 memoir, written with Sidney Shalett, describes the trip as a "rollicking fishing cruise into Southern waters," completely removing Dr. Heiter from the narrative, just as he had done for the 1933 assassination attempt.[45] The book also implies he attended his father's Easter service, even though he had left the ship in the Bahamas for Palm Beach the previous day and was summoned again to the yacht only after his father took ill. A page and a half is devoted to a fictional tale about Elliott—that his brother had flown to *Nourmahal* uninvited and nursing a hangover. Jimmy had flown to the anchorage with his brother. All of the travels of Jimmy and Elliott during this incident are well documented in newspaper articles and the deck log of the *Ellis*.[46,47,48]

The cruise was extended when radiation treatment brought about an unexpected medical emergency. The most likely scenario is supported by a mountain of evidence—the McEuen telegram, followed by a plethora of urgent secretive communications, Dr. Heiter's "duty" letter to his father on April 3, Marvin McIntyre's "Robbie was really very, very ill" letter—and, of course, the cover-ups by Franklin's two sons.

Franklin's fourth *Nourmahal* cruise was to see the America's Cup races off Newport, Rhode Island, over Labor Day weekend 1934. Doctor Heiter was invited but did not attend.[49] His fifth and last voyage took place between March 27 and April 7, 1935. Radiograms are found in FDR Library files

---

Worth on May 9. Hearst had taken a faster route to reconnect with Jimmy, flying to Texas from Los Angeles.

45 Roosevelt and Shalett, 280.

46 Jimmy's whereabouts are well documented. He had come to Florida on March 18 with his wife, Betsey, to vacation at Joseph P. Kennedy's Palm Beach Estate, attended a charity event for crippled children in Palm Beach on March 22 (*Palm Beach Post*, March 23, 1934). He joined his father in Jacksonville on March 28 "unexpectedly" deciding to sail at the last minute. He departed *Nourmahal* on the afternoon of March 30 (the day prior to the Easter service) by seaplane and was met in Miami by Betsey to return to Palm Beach. (*Palm Beach Post*, April 1, 1934) After Franklin became ill, he went back to Miami to join Elliott on April 3 for the seaplane flight to *Ellis*. Elliott returned on the seaplane after only a few hours, gave a news conference then proceeded to Washington with George Hearst. Jimmy remained aboard the yacht until it docked in Miami on April 11. None of this appears in his memoir.

47 A debt of thanks is due Jan Herman, who traveled to National Archives at College Park to examine the *Ellis* log on July 18, 2022.

48 It is unclear whether Franklin was transferred to *Ellis* for treatment. If that was the case Elliott was never aboard *Nourmahal*.

49 Heiter's son said the reason his father could not attend was that he could not afford the train fare. Phone call with the author.

from the Bahamas, but the "day by day" calendar states he was in Florida. "On this [trip], in addition to the President and me were Lytle Hull, [later to marry Vincent's first wife, Helen], Jimmy Roosevelt, Les Heiter, George St. George, W.R. Stewart, Frederic Kernochan and Kermit Roosevelt," Astor wrote to Grace Tully in 1949. "While in the Bahamas, Bede Clifford, the governor of the Bahamas, brought on board the King of England's youngest brother, Prince George, who subsequently became the Duke of Kent, and his very beautiful wife, Marina. The Duke of Kent was killed in the war."[50]

Dr. Heiter had returned to Alabama in 1931 to serve the people of Mobile—practicing surgery, general medicine and, primarily, obstetrics—working long hours mostly for barter or a nominal fee. Other than a few cruises aboard *Nourmahal*, Heiter put the lifestyle of the rich and famous behind him. There is no evidence he saw FDR again after 1935, but he continued to correspond with his friend Vincent Astor, who visited him in Alabama a few times as late as 1952. His only child, Bill, was born in 1945. Dr. Heiter died in 1979 at age 75, after a series of heart attacks.

---

50 Vincent Astor to Grace Tully, June 28, 1949, during preparation of her memoir. Grace Tully Papers, FDRL, Box 1.

■ Chapter 15

■ Settling In

Franklin's daily White House routine began at 8 a.m. with breakfast, while scanning *The New York Times, New York Herald Tribune, Washington Post and Herald, Baltimore Sun,* and *The Atlanta Constitution,* followed by a shave and haircut from his valet, Irving McDuffie.[1] This interlude also included a visit from White House physician Ross McIntire, briefings by members of his inner circle, a massage by George Fox, and other measures to enhance his appearance, especially of his left eye. The President rarely left his bedroom before 10 a.m.

The "day by day" calendar reveals a steady increase in the number of afternoon visits to the White House doctor's office beginning in 1934.[2,3] After 1939, no day went by without at least two medical visits. Daily treatments for Franklin's "sinus" problems almost surely included cocaine, an astringent and local anesthetic that had come into use in the 1880s. By the 1930s, the drug had become an important part of the therapeutic arsenal of head, eye, ear, nose, and throat (HEENT) specialists like McIntire.[4]

Franklin was nominated by acclamation at the 1936 Democratic National Convention in Philadelphia.[5] His acceptance speech was delivered at the University of Pennsylvania's Franklin Field before an audience of 100,000. The mood was triumphant. Conductor Leopold Stokowski led an orchestra

---

1 McDuffie had previously been a professional barber and began as FDR's valet in 1927. In 1939, he was "reassigned" by Eleanor after leaving the President unattended one morning following a bout of drinking. He died in 1946. His wife Lizzie remained employed as a maid at both the White House and Warm Springs and was present at FDR's death.

2 FDR Day by Day" is an exceedingly valuable and easily accessible tool to monitor much of Franklin's time as president, especially while he was in Washington. It is by no means complete and is clearly filtered to exclude much of his medical treatment, other than generic visits to the "doctor's office."

3 A search for "doctor's office" in Franklin's daily calendar reveals 5 visits in 1935, 7 in 1936 and 1937, 28 in 1938 and 234 in 1939.

4 Brain, P.F., Coward, G.A., "A Review of the History, Actions, and Legitimate Uses of Cocaine." *Journal of Substance Abuse* 1989;1(4):431–451. The drug was "discovered" in America by iconic surgeon William Stewart Halsted. It was used on Ulysses S. Grant to ease the pain of his terminal throat cancer in 1885.

5 The last presidential candidate to be so nominated was William Henry Harrison in 1840.

in "Hail to the Chief" as Franklin "walked" into view with James at his side. Spotlights illuminated his progress to the speaker's podium.

While on his way, Franklin was transferring his cane to his left hand to shake poet Edwin Markham's hand when a pin in the brace enclosing his left knee came loose. As he began to fall, his bodyguard, Gus Gennerich, caught him from behind before he could hit the floor.[6] The speech slipped from James's hand and the pages scattered. Secret Servicemen surrounded him to conceal the situation.

"There I was, hanging in the air like a goose about to be plucked," Franklin later told *Chicago Tribune* White House correspondent Walter Trohan, "but I kept on waving and smiling, and smiling and waving. I called to Jimmy out of the corner of my mouth to fix the pin. 'Dad,' Jimmy called up, 'I'm trying to pick up the speech.' 'To hell with the speech,' I said, again from the corner of my mouth. 'Fix the God-damned brace. If it can't be fixed there won't be any speech.' But I didn't lose a smile or a wave ... I could feel Jimmy fumbling and then I heard the pin snap back into place. My balance was restored and the weight was lifted from poor Gus."[7]

The anti-Roosevelt *Chicago Tribune* did not print the story of the stumble until thirty years after FDR's death. Such was the silence among reporters and photographers covering the Roosevelt White House. Journalists who tried to break the unwritten rule and show Franklin's handicap were "deterred" by the Secret Service. With one minor exception—a photo in *Life* magazine of Franklin in his wheelchair taken from a distance—no such image was published during his lifetime.[8]

Franklin took more than 60 percent of the popular vote in 1936, carrying every state except Maine and Vermont—winning the Electoral College by 523 to Republican Governor of Kansas Alf Landon's 8. "The test of our progress is not whether we add more to the abundance of those who have much," Franklin declared in his second inaugural address on January 20, 1937. "It is whether we provide enough for those who have too little."

---

6 Franklin had a deep affection for former New York State policeman Gus Gennerich, who died unexpectedly of a heart attack at age 50 while dancing at a restaurant during Franklin's trip to Argentina. Numerous handwritten letters by FDR mourn his passing.

7 Trohan, W., *Political Animals*. New York: Doubleday, 1975, 82–83.

8 Franklin was making a visit to the old Naval Hospital at Foggy Bottom to visit Interior Secretary Harold Ickes, who was recovering from a heart attack.

Louis Howe's death in April 1936 robbed Franklin of his most skilled political adviser. Other than Missy LeHand, only Howe could tell him to his face that he was wrong. Emboldened by his landslide victory, Franklin decided to flex his political muscles. In February 1937, the White House announced, without advance notice, a bill to expand the number of justices sitting on Supreme Court. The move angered politicians on both sides of the aisle. The legislation was soundly rejected by members of Congress even before it came up for a vote —the first dent in Franklin's shield of invincibility.

On August 5, 1937, Franklin signed Senate Bill No. 2067, which established a National Cancer Institute (NCI) in his own backyard at Bethesda, Maryland. At the dedication of the NCI's first building on October 31, 1940, he said: "The work of this new Institute is well under way. It is promoting and stimulating cancer research throughout the nation; it is bringing to the people of the nation a message of hope because many forms of the disease are not only curable but even preventable. Beyond this, it is doing research here and in many universities to unravel the mysteries of cancer. I think we can all have faith in the ultimate results of these great efforts."

Not every medical crisis was due to cancer. On November 16, 1937, Franklin was confined to bed with an abscessed tooth in his right lower jaw. "It is in Number 3 hole, aft, on the starboard side," he joked to reporters on November 23. The tooth had been extracted on November 17. Despite the availability of sulfa antibiotics, the infection hung on. "You don't look like a sick man, Mr. President," a reporter said at a November 26 press conference. "It is coming along all right," Franklin quipped. "I lost pounds and pounds." Three days later, he set out for the Caribbean on the presidential yacht *Potomac* for a week of fishing by day and poker by night.

"The President had been ill by an abscessed tooth, the drawing of which was too much delayed," Assistant Attorney General Robert Jackson wrote in a confidential memo. "It had caused a temperature running up to 103, had confined him to bed for several days, and resulted in a general upset ... [on the way from Washington to Miami], the President was not in high spirits, his jaw was visibly swollen. There was not the customary quickness of reaction. By December 1 he was feeling decidedly better."[9]

---

9 Jackson, R.H., *That Man: An Insider's Portrait of Franklin D. Roosevelt.* Oxford: Oxford University Press, 2003, 142–143.

Another shipmate, Interior Secretary Harold Ickes, had a similar observation: "I was a good deal worried about the President on this trip ... he didn't seem at all like himself. He looked bad and seemed listless, he kept very much to himself," Ickes wrote. "Even when he was out on deck ... he seemed to have the appearance of a man who has more or less given up. Towards the end of the trip he acted much better which led me to the conclusion that he had been showing the effects of his bad tooth. All of the time that we were away some of the infection from the tooth was still present. This was the reason Dr. McIntire finally persuaded him to cut the trip a couple of days short and return to Washington."[10]

Discussion of the tooth infection was permitted at the press conference in Miami on December 5.

Q: How do you feel?

THE PRESIDENT: Well, it is still there ... I don't know the medical term. Putting it as a layman, I would say that it has not healed and if it does not heal very quickly, they will probably curette it. I don't even know how to spell it. How do you spell it, Ross?

DR. McINTIRE: Scrape would be better.

THE PRESIDENT: They will scrape the bone.

DR. McINTIRE: It just has not healed up the way we think it should so we think we had better get back to where it can be looked over.

Q: Have you been running any temperature?

THE PRESIDENT: I haven't except for this. It is still sore.

A given voyage's guest list and vessel are good clues to a particular trip's purpose. This late November sail included Jackson and Ickes—neither of whom were privy to Franklin's innermost health secrets—and took place aboard *Potomac*, nowhere near *Nourmahal's* nor any warship's league as a floating medical facility.

---

10 *Secret Diary of Harold Ickes.* New York: Simon & Schuster, January 1954, Entry for December 6, 1937. Ickes' diaries are a valuable historical record. The later years are only available on microfilm at the FDR Library.

■ Chapter 16
■ Camouflage

A cancer diagnosis in the 1930s was akin to one for AIDS in the 1980s. Doctors labeled fear of the disease "cancerphobia." It was believed by the lay public to be infectious and hereditary—an illness to be kept under wraps. Family members lobbied to falsify cancer patients' death certificates. Even a hint Franklin had the disease would have torpedoed his political career.

The author's peer-reviewed 2008 paper with iconic dermatologist A. Bernard Ackerman narrowed the differential diagnosis of Franklin's pigmented lesion to two—melanoma and a benign "age spot" known scientifically as seborrheic keratosis, neither of which is known to shrink, in clinical terms, "regress," as rapidly as Franklin's growth did. The *only* explanation for the lesion's disappearance is surgical removal. "I'm not stating unequivocally that he had melanoma," Ackerman told ABC News in 2008. "But it sure looks like it."

Due to the complicity of the press and a long stream of adulatory pieces in *Liberty* magazine, Franklin's health was no longer an impediment to a run for a third term, though efforts to soften the appearance, if not the mortal threat, of the cancer were ongoing. A series of minor operations were performed, timed for a brief enough recovery to avoid raising suspicion. Just how many is deeply hidden but photographs and newsreel footage document a sequential surgical removal. Some images reveal surgical scars and remnants of suture material. Most evident, though, is Ross McIntire's skill as a plastic surgeon.

The earliest concrete evidence of surgical treatment after Dr. Heiter's 1933 operation aboard *Nourmahal* is in a March 1937 issue of *Life* in which the caption of a photo taken at Warm Springs mentioned Franklin undergoing treatment for a "sty."

> "President Roosevelt uses his fingers on a piece of fried chicken at a barbeque in Warm Springs, Ga. The President is getting his second helping from Love Terry, waitress. The day before the barbeque Mr. Roosevelt emerged from a four-day retirement at the 'Little White House,' spent nursing a sty on his eye and avoiding photographers."

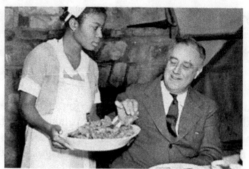

March 1937 Life magazine pjoto of FDR after his
operation for a "sty" above his left eye.

"A sty in his *left* eye, three days of intermittent rain and cold at Warm Springs, Ga., and bad weather that grounded a plane carrying official mail, contrived last week to give Franklin Roosevelt as much rest as even a President could desire," *Time* reported on March 29. Both the setting and the time frame are consistent with the modus operandi of the cover-up. FDR had undergone one of his minor operations. An operating suite, mostly for orthopedic procedures, was part of the Warm Springs medical facility.

Franklin's doctors pushed therapeutic and cosmetic limits of surgery and radiation to their limits. A search for alternative options led to an early form of immunotherapy. William B. Coley had been a founder of the New York Cancer Hospital, in 1916 renamed the Memorial Hospital for Cancer and Allied Diseases,[1] and was that facility's chief of orthopedics until 1933. In the 1880s, Coley observed that cancers sometimes shrank in patients who had developed fevers caused by bacterial infections.[2] As an experiment, Coley deliberately infected cancer patients. After disastrous results with live bacteria, he began using denatured, noninfectious material and arrived at a regimen that appeared to shrink several tumor types, including melanomas.[3,4] "Coley's

---

1 Since 1960, the Memorial Sloane Kettering Cancer Center. https://www.mskcc.org/about/history-milestones.

2 In particular, *Serratia Marcescens.*

3 Coley, W.B., "The Treatment of Malignant Tumors by Repeated Inoculations of Erysipelas: With a Report of Ten Original Cases." *Clinical Orthopaedics and Related Research* 1893 May;105:487–511.

4 For a succinct, entertaining review of the topic of Coley and his Toxins, see the excellent article by Matt Castle at https:///www.damninteresting.com/coley's-cancer-killing-concoction/. For a more comprehensive treatment see: McCarthy, E.F., "The Toxins of

Toxins," as the substance came to be called, gained a following and Parke Davis Pharmaceuticals began manufacturing it commercially in the late 1890s. As new therapies with x-ray and radium took hold and radical surgery became less risky, Coley's Toxins lost favor but remained in limited use until the arrival of chemotherapy in the 1950s.[5,6]

A cancer patient typically reacts to this form of immunotherapy with a few days of low-grade fever. Franklin's daily White House calendar lists at least five instances of a "slight cold" accompanied by fever between September 1933 and March 1941, each beginning on Sunday and lasting two days.[7] Another began the day after Christmas. The pattern is beyond coincidence and makes a strong case Franklin was treated with Coley's Toxins. Whether or not the use of this novel treatment extended Franklin's life is debatable, but Franklin survived with melanoma for fifteen years before succumbing to the disease, far longer than would have been statistically expected.

A May 22, 1939, photo shows a fresh surgical scar above Franklin's left eye as well as a small lesion below the larger growth that would soon disappear.[8]

William B. Coley and the Treatment of Bone and Soft-Tissue Sarcomas." *Iowa Orthopedic Journal* 2006;26:154–158.

5 As understanding of the immune response advanced, the active component of Coley's Toxins, a protein, tumor necrosis factor alpha, was discovered in 1975.

6 For more information about Coley's Toxins and the feud between Coley and James Ewing as to their use, see: https://chipsahospital.org/dr-james-ewing-vs-dr-william-coley-how-cancer-might-be-cured/ (last accessed October 31, 2022).

7 FDR Day by Day, FDRL.

8 Archives of Harris and Ewing photographers.

Favorable camera angles and photo retouching were successful in deflecting public attention from the melanoma until January 1940, the White House received a letter from Massachusetts cancer specialist Dr. Reuben Peterson expressing his concern about the growth over the president's eye. Ross McIntire's reply on January 25, 1940, is the only written acknowledgment of the lesion's existence. "I will say to you in confidence that the pigmented area above the President's eye is very superficial and has never shown any sign of an inflammatory nature," McIntire wrote to Peterson. "You can rest assured it is under observation at all times."[9] A photograph taken on January 30, 1940, reveals two long horizontal scars within the eyebrow. The oval-shaped primary lesion has expanded through the first horizontal skinfold above the eyebrow and below its lower margin.[10]

On August 16, 1940, Franklin donned a blue seersucker suit and plaid tie and was wheeled into the Oval Office for photographers from the capital's leading studios—Harris & Ewing, Underwood, and Hessler. An unpublished Hessler Studios proof provides irrefutable evidence that the area over Roosevelt's left eye had undergone changes attributable only to surgical intervention. A piece of suture material is seen over the eye and sparse hairs are combed over a long scar within the base of the eyebrow. The primary lesion appears lighter, with less distinct margins than the deep brown spot seen in film and photographs taken six months earlier during Franklin's trip to Panama aboard *Tuscaloosa*.

9 Ross McIntire to Reuben Peterson (retained copy), January 25, 1940, Ross McIntire papers, FDRL.
10 Archives of Harris and Ewing photographers.

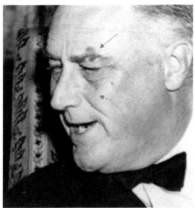

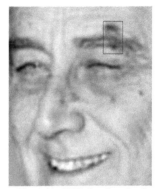

May 22, 1939 photo of FDR showing fresh surgical scar.

Close-up FDR in the Oval Office showing retained suture material, August 16, 1940.

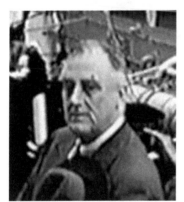

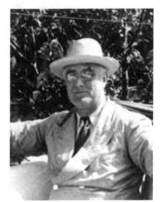

August 1940 photos of FDR showing extent of growth of pigmented lesion in above and below left eyebrow.

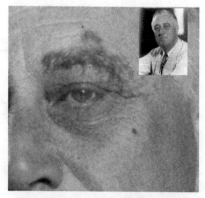

One of the two small pigmented lesions below the left eye had been removed—subtle yet unequivocal evidence of surgical removal.

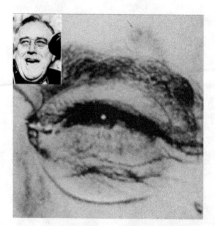

A photo taken through a telephoto lens at the dedication of New York City's Queens Midtown Tunnel on October 28, shows a circular scar where the stray piece of suture had been in August.

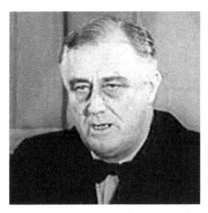

By the "Arsenal of Democracy" speech on December 27, the lesion was just a shadow.

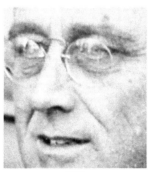
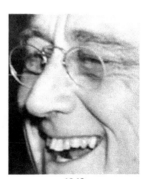

 1933

1942

By March 1942 visible evidence of the growth had been almost completely erased, though Dr. Heiter's 1932 surgical scar remained.

■ Chapter 17
■ To Run or Not to Run

As 1940 approached, Franklin was keeping his options open regarding retirement, including plans for a library at Springwood to house his books as well as documents and mementos from his time in office (the Presidential Records Act was not passed until 1978).[1]

At the annual Gridiron Dinner in December 1939, a skit lampooned Franklin's shilly-shallying about a third term. The centerpiece was a papier-mâché Sphinx with the president's face and trademark cigarette holder—a three-dimensional version of what many a newspaper editorial cartoon had likened him to—the mythical Egyptian creature that forever posed a riddle it refused to answer.

The Roosevelt family was opposed to a run. "Mother and every one of us felt that Father had done his job, had done it well, and that he deserved a rest," son James wrote. "Frankly, we didn't want to lose him." Most evidence prior to mid-1940 suggests Franklin tended to agree. On January 17, he signed a $175,000 ($3,700,000 in 2022) contract with *Collier's* magazine to write a series of articles over three years, introducing editor William Cheyney around the White House as his "future boss"—not what might be expected of a leader anticipating four more years as President.

"Missy told Jane [Ickes] that the President is very tired and was really looking forward to retiring at the end of the year," Harold Ickes wrote on January 27, 1940. "[Jane] wants the President to run again … the latter told Missy that 'God will provide a candidate.' [Missy's] retort was that God had better get busy pretty soon."

Joseph P. Kennedy asked Franklin about a third term in December 1939. "I can't. I'm tired. I can't take it," he responded. "What I need is a year's rest. I just won't go for a third term unless we are in war. Even then, I'll never send an army over. We'll help them but with supplies."

---

1 The idea of a library came from Missy LeHand.

When Labor Secretary Frances Perkins suggested future policies to Franklin, he chuckled, then quipped, "Don't you know I'm through in January 1941?" or "You will have to speak with the next President about that." Shortly after Christmas 1939, Perkins brought Teamsters Union president Daniel J. Tobin for an evening meeting in the second-floor White House oval study. "You just *have* to run for the third term," Tobin said. "Don't talk to me about your fishing trips next winter—you are going to be right here in the White House."

"No, Dan," Franklin responded, "I just can't do it. I tell you, I have been here a long time. I am tired. I really am. You don't know what it's like. And besides, I have to take care of myself. I never had it until I came here. How can I get over it? This sinus trouble I've got, the Washington climate made it dreadful. The doctors say I have to go into the hospital for a month of steady treatment. But I can't do that, you know. When a President does that, the bottom drops out of the stock market, the Japs take advantage of what they think is a serious illness, the Germans start propaganda that I am dying and that the United States is in a panic. No, I can't be president again. I have to get over this sinus. I have to have a rest. I want to go home to Hyde Park. I want to take care of my trees ... finish my little house on the hill ... write history. No, I just can't do it, Dan."[2]

When Nebraska Senator George Norris visited the White House to urge Franklin to run for a third term, FDR expressed remarkably candid frustration with his immobility: "George, I am chained to this chair from morning 'til night. People come in here day after day most of them trying to get something from me, most of them things I can't give them, and I wouldn't if I could. You sit in your chair in your office too, but if something goes wrong or you get irritated or tired, you can get up and walk around, or you can go into another room. But I can't. I am tied down to this chair day after day week after week month after month and I can't stand it any longer. I can't go on with it."[3]

In January 1940, Harry Hopkins was "virtually certain" Franklin would run. By April 23 he had grave doubts. "The President seemed disinclined to [do] anything about the nomination or permit any of his friends to do anything, which would have meant it would go to the [Jim] Farley faction by default," Hopkins told Robert Sherwood.[4]

---

2 Perkins, 126.
3 Morgan, T., *FDR: A Biography*. New York: Simon & Schuster, 1985, 519–520.
4 Sherwood, R., *Roosevelt and Hopkins*. New York: Harper and Brothers, 1948, 172.

Franklin's resolve to leave office had likely been hardened by ongoing medical problems. On January 10, radiologist Charles F. Behrens interpreted a sinus x-ray as revealing "haziness in the frontal sinus and swelling of the nasal passages *on one side*."[5] Secrecy about the cancer was so tight that Behrens was not permitted to document in writing which side of Franklin's head was affected.

On February 10, Franklin passed out at dinner with Missy and her romantic interest, Ambassador William Bullitt—most likely from severe pain. Earlier in the day he had spent an hour with a dentist and an additional hour in the doctor's office. Ross McIntire wrote off the episode as a "mild heart attack."[6] The next day's calendar is blank until a 4:30 p.m. meeting, followed by a 90-minute conference to discuss strategy for averting American entry into the war with Under Secretary of State Sumner Welles, who was heading off to Europe for talks with leaders there.

On February 13 Franklin announced he would be taking a "vacation" with limited press access—a reliable indicator that a medical problem was about to be addressed. "I am going to leave tomorrow and take a little trip of about ten days," he told reporters. "I don't know definitely yet what port I am going from. I am going to get on a boat and that is why I am going to limit it to the three press associations."

"President Decides on Vacation at Sea in Air of Mystery," The *New York Times* headlined on February 13. "Vague on Details of Trip to Start Today— Seems Weary as He Tells Press of Plan." Reporters followed the President on a destroyer convoy. "Their dispatches would be censored, as usual, by the President himself. Neither from the President nor other White House sources was there any explanation for the unusual secrecy with which his movements are being surrounded," the *Times* reported.

The next day, Franklin, Ross McIntire, "Pa" Watson, and naval aide Captain Daniel Callaghan[7] entrained for Pensacola, Florida, where heavy cruiser USS

---

5 Charles Francis Behrens was the radiologist charged with interpreting FDR's x-rays from 1940 until his death. Early radiologists were both diagnostic and therapeutic. Any radiation therapy given to FDR would have been overseen by him as well. Behrens edited *Atomic Medicine* in 1949, the first textbook on the subject.

6 McIntire did not diagnose a "heart attack" in the context of thrombosis of a coronary artery, but rather, in this case, as a generic description of passing out due to a cardiovascular cause, basically a fainting spell.

7 Callaghan was killed in action on the bridge of his ship during the battle of Savo Island (Guadalcanal) on November 13, 1942.

Tuscaloosa was waiting. Franklin had been aboard previously for a sail to Campobello in 1939.[8]

The "mystery cruise," as the press labeled it,[9] was billed by the White House as an inspection of Panama Canal defenses. Franklin met with local dignitaries and fished from the cruiser's deck, but the trip was almost surely another of his maritime escapes for medical treatment. "Have had no word from you. Hope all goes well," Missy anxiously telexed from Washington on February 16. Two days later Franklin responded, "All well. Good trip." [10]

The day prior to disembarking, Franklin gave a brief speech to thank the cruiser's crew. Captain Harry A. Badt ended his short introduction, "The officers and men of the *Tuscaloosa* all want to wish you continued good health."[11]

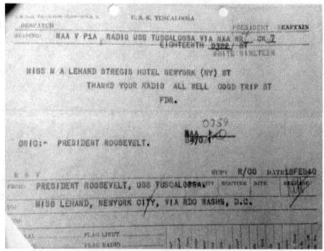

Telegram from FDR to Missy Lehand from USS Tuscalsoosa during the mystery cruise.

---

8 His last visit to the family vacation home.
9 "President Decides on Vacation at Sea in Air of Mystery." *New York Times*, February 13, 1940.
10 Trips of the President.
11 He would make a third and final cruise aboard the *Tuscaloosa* in December with Harry Hopkins to work out the details of Lend-Lease.

The procedure performed on the "mystery cruise" was most likely to treat yet another of Franklin's medical problems—prostate cancer. A large body of evidence—FBI memoranda, the Suckley diary, doctors interviewed by Harry Goldsmith, the urologist's daughter, and even an admission by Eleanor Roosevelt that her husband had the disease, makes a strong circumstantial case that Franklin was diagnosed with prostate cancer in 1940 and suffered its consequences until his death.

No form of cancer affects more men than cancer of the prostate, a gland which produces the fluid that transports semen. One man in nine is diagnosed with the disease. Left untreated, prostate cancer can obstruct the flow of urine and metastasize most notoriously—and painfully—to the bones of the hips, pelvis, and lower spine. There is circumstantial evidence, especially from the Suckley diary, that this is what happened to FDR.

Treatment for cancer of the prostate in 1940 was limited to surgically removing the gland or burning out the tumor with radiation. Since 1915, doctors had been using a procedure known as brachytherapy[12] to treat the disease—inserting radium-tipped needles into a patient's prostate gland for several hours through the skin of the perineum, the region between the anus and the testicular sac.[13] After a few days, the irradiated area predictably becomes inflamed and swollen, causing intense discomfort lasting "a number of days to some weeks."[14] For comfort and to ensure unobstructed flow of urine, doctors often fit brachytherapy patients with a urinary catheter.

Franklin returned to Washington from his "mystery cruise" on March 2 and maintained a full calendar of appointments for a little over a week. But on March 11, Steve Early announced the president was "confined to the house with intestinal flu." Franklin had probably been sidelined by the delayed effects of brachytherapy.

The cover story was a purely fictional diagnosis, "swamp fever."[15] "He was preparing to come to the office when Dr. McIntire came in and took his temperature," Early told reporters on March 15, "The President was achy and grippy

---

12 The word is derived from the Latin *brachus*, meaning short distance.
13 Janeway, H.H., Barringer, B.S., *Radium Therapy in Cancer at the Memorial Hospital New York*. New York: Paul B. Hoeber, 1917, 233–237.
14 *Ibid.*
15 There is no such disease. The name came from the collective imaginations of Early, McIntire, and FDR.

and had a degree of temperature. It is a continuation or holdover of the condition that kept him at the house for four or five days earlier this week." At McIntire's behest, Early added, Franklin was confined to the White House and had canceled his press conference, his Cabinet meeting, and all other engagements—likely catheterized and tethered to an icepack. Needing entertainment, he convened reporters on March 19. Usually forbidden questions about his health were permitted.

REPORTER: "How are you feeling?"

FDR: "Rotten. I ache still. It's the old flu."

REPORTER: "Still hangs on?"

FDR: "Yes, I thought I would come over here and try it instead of sitting upstairs."

REPORTER: "Do you think you will go away?"

FDR: "I do not know. I will be going to Warm Springs as soon as I can."

Later that day, Harold Ickes paid Franklin a sickroom visit to encourage him to run for a third term. "Suppose I should become so ill that I could not possibly be a candidate?" Franklin asked.

"You oughtn't to talk like that!" Ickes retorted.

Ickes returned on March 25, afterwards confiding to his diary, "He has been laid up for ten days following a light attack of intestinal flu but has not been able to get rid of the temperature."

On March 26, fifteen days after the original announcement, Early announced, "The doctor does not think it advisable, yet, to throw the president into a press conference, so we are cancelling the conference today as a purely precautionary measure."

REPORTER: How is the old "swamp fever"? Any temperature?

EARLY: No, he is quite all right. Ross thinks it is a question of keeping him in the same environment and not changing it so much. So, he is remaining at the House today.

REPORTER: Is the Warm Springs trip shaping up any more, Steve?

EARLY: It has not been mentioned.

REPORTER: The newspaper boys seem to think he is going away the latter part of the week.

EARLY: I think it is just a hope. I don't think it will be in the earlier part or the latter part of the week.

REPORTER: That kind of narrows it down. You sound like a politician.

EARLY: I got that out of the old seventh chapter by J. Russell Young on how to be obscure when the need exists.[16]

By now, Franklin, McIntire, and Early could have written the book about being obscure.

On March 28, *The New York Times* reported Franklin had now "completely recovered from the cold which has kept him from his desk in the last few weeks." He resumed a limited schedule the next day.

Ickes wrote on April 5 that Franklin told him his temperature had been normal for two days but the intestinal flu had left him with gas in his colon, so he had "given up the idea of going to Warm Springs." The President acted "well and hearty," Ickes wrote, but still showed the effects of his illness. "Swamp fever" had now flip-flopped to a "cold" that was "much better."

Laboratory reports offer clues to what was ailing Franklin. A chest x-ray, using one of Franklin's more inventive aliases, "Andrew Jackson," revealed chronic lung irritation—not surprising for a two-pack-a-day Camel smoker.[17] On March 21, his white blood cell count was elevated at 13,900, an indication of the body fighting infection or inflammation. On March 23, that figure was 12,400; by March 27 it was a normal 9,200. Neutrophils, a specific type of white blood cell linked to inflammation, were mildly elevated. Hemoglobin level (a reflection of the amount of red blood cells) was normal at 13.5. A test for bacteria in the blood was negative. Stool analysis revealed the presence of *Entamoeba Coli*, a benign single-celled parasite. A urinalysis, potentially the most revealing test since the most probable source of inflammation was in the urinary tract, is suspiciously absent.

---

16 Young was the dean of the White House Press Corps.

17 The report read: "diffuse fibrosis probably consequent chronic tracheo-bronchitis" and "no infiltrative pathology of the tubercular type. There is a mottled increased density about the right main bronchus suggestive of residuals of a small patch of central pneumonitis."

Fevers of this duration do not usually accompany a viral illness like flu or the common cold.[18] The laboratory results are consistent with a relatively mild inflammatory process. Irritation of the prostate gland and urinary bladder from radiation is high on the list of possibilities.

To squelch rumors still swirling in Washington about Franklin's illness, *Liberty* magazine ran an article in the May 18 issue under the provocative title "Is President Roosevelt Fit for a Third Term?" The story addressed "swamp fever" head-on. "A few weeks ago President Roosevelt cancelled his press conference and appointments and took himself to bed with what everyone assumed to be another one of his colds," journalist Walter Karig wrote. The usual period of rest and isolation passed, but the President did not resume his office routine. Officials with whom business had to be transacted were summoned to his bedroom. Rear Admiral Ross McIntire, Mr. Roosevelt's personal physician, informed the White House newspaper correspondents through Stephen Early that an intermittent fever of one degree or less was hanging on stubbornly.

> "With his few visitors the president joked about his 'touch of swamp fever.' These visitors, waylaid by the press, declared that he did not look sick or act so at all. But when he delayed his long projected visit to Warm Springs, Georgia, gossip flared. One heard fantastic stories in the corners and corridors of the Capitol. It was solemnly asserted as the real inside dope that the president, informed he could not survive a third term, was going to seek reelection anyhow.

> "Perhaps all the rumors could have been prevented if full frankness had prevailed. Franklin D. Roosevelt is a mortal man with a stomach and kidneys and intestines and lungs that get out of order occasionally like anybody else's. What ailed him in April was a mild intestinal influenza."

> "I think that for a man of fifty-eight the President is certainly in as good health as we could expect anybody to be," Dr. McIntire told Karig. "Notable among these is his remarkable physical reserve, his immense power of recuperation. The rest of us on the White House staff would be dead if we had to keep pace with him."

---

18 One possible scenario for the timing of onset of symptoms and the protracted recovery could be inflammation of the prostate following treatment with radium-needle brachytherapy on the *Tuscaloosa* in February. It would also explain the fever and the protracted absence from the public. Such a procedure causes frequent, painful urination, including the possibility of catheterization, as well as torturous discomfort with prolonged sitting, something the wheelchair-bound President could not avoid.

"Roosevelt has something that no other president in my time has had," John Russell Young, dean of the White House press corps, is quoted as saying. "That is a God-sent gift which enables him to lock up all his tremendous worries and responsibilities in some mental cupboard ... and forget them while he relaxes in pure fun. Then he unlocks the cupboard, hauls out the grim business of being president, and tackles the job, mentally refreshed." The article continues with columns of blather about Franklin's superhuman behavior.

Franklin and Missy escaped to Warm Springs on April 16, where Canadian Prime Minister Mackenzie King paid him a visit. "[Franklin] repeated to me he did not intend to have a third term," King confided to his diary. "I sought to impress upon him to keep in mind his health and strength. That to attempt anything which might mean a breakdown in his own health would be to imperil, for the future, much of the work that he had performed and which he could oversee in a quiet way if giving his time, for example, to writing, etc. I studied him pretty closely as we were together."

> "I found him frankly better in appearance than I had expected to see him. Not so exhausted. He was much thinner in body. Tells me he has lost ten pounds; also in the face, but not haggard or worn looking, though eyes very tired. I noted too he seemed to be inwardly quite nervous at times and showed real fatigue ... Miss LeHand, with whom I spoke privately, seemed to share a like view. Dr. McIntire thought physically he was in good shape and could stand a third term should he attempt it. Personally, I do not think he should."[19]

On May 10, British Prime Minister Neville Chamberlain, dying of cancer, resigned after losing a vote of confidence in the House of Commons.[20] Leadership of the British Empire was assumed by a sixty-five-year-old, chain-smoking, alcoholic former First Lord of the Admiralty—Winston Spencer Churchill. That summer, Churchill's stirring rhetoric and dramatic radio reports from blitz-torn London by CBS reporters Edward R. Murrow and Robert Trout went a long way toward convincing Americans of the necessity to assist Hitler's enemies—but at this point the voters' main question was still whether or not their President was going to run a third time.

Performing a balancing act between an urgent need to bolster America's depleted, antiquated armed forces and strong isolationist sentiment, Franklin addressed a joint session of Congress to appeal for $1.2 billion ($25.5 billion

---

19 *Diary of Mackenzie King.* Ottawa: Library and Archives Canada, 2006, April 23–24, 1940.
20 Chamberlain died exactly six months later.

in 2022) for "defense" on May 16, 1940. "Our objective is still peace—peace at home and peace abroad," he said, "Nevertheless, we stand ready not only to spend millions for defense but to give our service and even our lives for the maintenance of our American liberties."

The best chronology of Franklin's journey of decision to run for a third term comes from speechwriter Sam Rosenman. "As late as February 1940 Hopkins talked to me about his own plan of buying a home and retiring in the neighborhood of Hyde Park," Rosenman wrote. "The President was building a hilltop cottage there for greater privacy. I was convinced during the Spring months of 1940 that the president—at least until the day that Norway was invaded [April 9]—was absolutely determined not to seek a third term … Until the violation of the neutrality act of Holland and Belgium and the invasion of France on May 10, he was somewhat in doubt. After Dunkirk [the evacuation ended on June 4, 1940], I am sure his mind was made up."[21]

The lead article in the June 10, 1940, issue of *Time* magazine revealed just how effective Franklin had been in protecting what speechwriter Robert Sherwood called his "heavily-forested interior."[22]

"The Mystery. Last week, Franklin Delano Roosevelt, 58 years old, seven generations removed from a Dutch settler of 1644, son of a country gentleman and the belle of the Hudson River valley, was head of the last great democracy still at peace, with 33 weeks left of his second term," *Time* wrote. "Yet, although he was in his eighth year as President, although he had moved, worked, eaten, laughed, exhorted, prayed in the intensest glare of public scrutiny, although his every facial grimace, the tone of his voice, each mannerism, *the dark mole over his left eyebrow (emphasis added)*, the mole on his right cheek—although all these were public property, intimate to every U.S. citizen, still there was no man in the United States who could answer the question, Who Is Franklin Roosevelt?"[23]

Franklin had been hounding Secretary of State Cordell Hull to be his running mate. On June 20, he gave him an ultimatum. "If you don't take it, I'll have to get Henry Wallace," "That's all right with me," Hull replied.[24]

---

21 Rosenman, 193.
22 Sherwood, 1948.
23 *Time*, June 10, 1940.
24 *Memoirs of Cordell Hull*. New York: Macmillan, 1948, 858–861.

Franklin met with Jim Farley on July 7 in Hyde Park. "I was convinced he had already made up his mind on Wallace and had determined not to disclose his choice until the last minute in order to keep the field of vice-presidential candidates in line for the third term," Farley wrote in his memoir. Quoting Franklin, he added, "'The man running with me must be in good health because there is no telling how long I can hold out. You know, Jim, a man with paralysis can have a breakup at any time. While my heart and lungs are good and the other organs functioning along okay, nothing in this life is certain.' With that, he pulled up his shirt, unbuttoned, and showed me a lump of flesh and muscle under his left shoulder, which he said were misplaced because of his affliction [polio]," Farley wrote. "He noted that he must sit most of the time. 'It's essential that the man who runs with me should be able to carry on,' tucking his shirt back in and reaching for another cigarette. It was the first and last time in all the years I knew him that he ever discussed his physical condition with me."[25]

The Democratic convention began in Chicago on July 15. Franklin remained in Washington, where Fulton Oursler, editor of *Liberty* magazine, witnessed a conversation at the White House about Montana Senator Burton K. Wheeler's opposition to American involvement in the war. "Sam Rosenman had come in to tell the President that Senator [Claude] Pepper was on the phone from the convention in Chicago," Oursler wrote. "I asked the President if he wanted me to retire. He said 'No.' It was now my privilege to listen to the President in one of the most towering rages that any man let himself get into without committing mayhem. 'All Senator Wheeler wants is to win a moral victory over me in the newspapers and you can tell him for me that I am not going to let him,' Franklin told Pepper. 'You tell Senatah Wheelah for me I can blast him out of the water.' At this point Rosenman got up and went out of the room. The President was panting heavily. I noticed a flap of flesh that had grown over his left eye [almost surely a skin graft from one of Ross McIntire's procedures] and other visible physical deteriorations, but also I told myself I had never seen him so aroused, so jumpy, so nervously unsettled."[26]

Franklin kept his decision about running close to the vest until the last moment to maintain a high level of tension. He did not want a roll call vote, preferring

---

25 *Jim Farley's Story*. Whittlesey House, 1948, 156. The book was ghost written by Walter Trohan. The original manuscript is in the Trohan papers at the Herbert Hoover Library, North Branch, Iowa.

26 Oursler, F., *Behold the Dreamer! An Autobiography*. New York: Little Brown, 1964, 438–440.

to be nominated by acclamation to ensure a united party behind him. The delegates included a substantial number of isolationists who had succeeded in having a plank inserted into the party platform declaring, "We will not participate in foreign wars and we will not send our army or navy or air force to fight in foreign lands outside of the Americas." The Roosevelt camp softened that language by tacking on "except in case of attack."[27]

Democratic national chairman Jim Farley controlled ticket distribution, so many in the galleries at Chicago Stadium were supporters of his presidential candidacy. But Franklin had a trick up his sleeve, a stunt he had worked out with Chicago Mayor Edward Kelly. The convention's keynote address was delivered by Senate Majority Leader Alben Barkley of Kentucky, a strong Roosevelt supporter. Barkley closed with "a message from the President." Franklin, he said, had no "desire or purpose to continue in the office of President, to be a candidate for that office, or to be nominated by the convention for that office. He wishes in all conviction and in sincerity to make it clear that all of the delegates ... are free to vote for any candidate."[28]

The disavowal stunned the delegates into silence. Suddenly, from loudspeakers around the hall came a voice chanting, "We want Roosevelt!" Simultaneously, the Chicago police department band marched in playing Franklin's 1932 campaign song "Happy Days Are Here Again," while the disembodied voice repeatedly shouted, "We want Roosevelt! Everybody wants Roosevelt! The world needs Roosevelt!" Delegates and spectators began to take up the chant.[29]

The invisible cheerleader was a Kelly stalwart, Chicago Sanitary District Superintendent Thomas D. Garry, later remembered as "the voice from the sewers." Franklin sailed to renomination with 946 votes to Farley's 72 and Vice President Garner's 61.

The Republican presidential nominee, Indiana businessman Wendell Willkie, had publicly agreed with Franklin that the United States had to be ready for war, eliminating any prospect of the GOP mining isolationists for support. When Congress considered instituting a military draft, Willkie supported the bill, which passed by a one vote majority. The principal issue in the election was whether Franklin, or anyone, should have a third term. But the nation was grateful that the President had led them through perilous times, and many

---

27 Smith, J.E., 458.
28 *Ibid.*, 460.
29 *Ibid.*

voters feared that an untested leader would not be a wise choice for a nation on the verge of war. In November, Franklin received his historic mandate to lead America for another four years, carrying 38 states with 449 electoral votes to Willkie's 82.

Chapter 18

"Pa Had Really Been Quite Ill"

Franklin sensed a need for unity and brought more Republicans into his new administration. He appointed Frank Knox, the GOP's vice-presidential nominee in 1936, as Secretary of the Navy and tapped Henry Stimson, Herbert Hoover's Secretary of State, to be Secretary of War. Stimson later remarked how Franklin "carried his burden with such buoyant courage."[1,2]

1941 began with the introduction of Franklin's most enduring credo. In the peroration of his State of the Union address on January 6, he announced:

> "In the future days, which we seek to make secure, we look forward to a world founded upon four essential human freedoms.
>
> "The first is freedom of speech and expression—everywhere in the world.
>
> "The second is freedom of every person to worship God in his own way—everywhere in the world.
>
> "The third is freedom from want—which, translated into world terms, means economic understandings which will secure to every nation a healthy peacetime life for its inhabitants—everywhere in the world.
>
> "The fourth is freedom from fear—which, translated into world terms, means a world-wide reduction of armaments to such a point and in such a thorough fashion that no nation will be in a position to commit an act of physical aggression against any neighbor—anywhere in the world.
>
> "That is no vision of a distant millennium," Franklin told a joint session of Congress, "It is a definite basis for a kind of world attainable in our own time and generation."

On March 11, Congress passed "Lend-Lease," a program conceived with Harry Hopkins to support Britain in its existential battle against Hitler, while

---

1 Gallagher, 169.

2 Harold Ickes had been a liberal Republican going back to the days of TR's Bull Moose party. Henry Wallace's roots began with the GOP. The short-lived Secretary of the Treasury, William Woodin, was a Republican businessman. Thanks to historian Derek Leebaert for pointing this out.

still maintaining the guise of American neutrality. The law permitted the United States to "sell, transfer title to, exchange, lease, lend, or otherwise dispose of, to any such government [whose defense the President deems vital to the defense of the United States] any defense article." In April, the policy was extended to China; in October, to the Soviet Union.

On May 4, Franklin traveled to the sleepy Shenandoah Valley town of Staunton, Virginia, to dedicate the newly restored boyhood home of Woodrow Wilson. The speech was to be followed by a tour of the local caverns.

The president seemed pale and listless. Unusually fatigued, he begged off spelunking and returned to Washington. The next morning, Lieutenant Commander George Adam Fox snapped into action. A career Navy man, Fox was Ross McIntire's right hand. Since 1933, no man had spent more private time with Franklin. Two decades earlier Fox had been the medical aide and masseur for the disabled Woodrow Wilson. Like McIntire and "Pa" Watson, Fox had come into Franklin's inner circle at the recommendation of Cary Grayson.[3] Aside from giving daily massages and coordinating presidential medications and testing, Fox, or possibly valet Arthur Prettyman,[4] likely assumed the role of makeup artist, going to the president's bedroom each morning to camouflage the surgical scarring over his left eye.

McIntire filled out a laboratory request for patient "F. David Rolph"—Franklin's medical aliases sometimes played on the initials "FDR." Fox drew up a few vials of blood and hand-carried them a little over a mile down Constitution Avenue NW to the naval hospital on the hill at Foggy Bottom.[5] McIntire must have gasped in disbelief as he saw the results and recognized that his patient had a life-threatening anemia—and it was he who was responsible. Franklin's hemoglobin level, a measure of the body's quantity of red blood cells, was 4.5 grams per liter, one-third of normal. The data also revealed that Franklin had been losing blood to internal bleeding for many months. In March 1940, his hemoglobin level had been normal. Since then, eight pints of blood had somehow seeped away.

---

3 Cary Grayson Papers, Staunton, VA.
4 Prettyman replaced Irwin McDuffie, after the latter abandoned FDR one evening during a drinking binge.
5 The Naval Hospital was located at the site of the old Naval observatory where the moons of Mars had been discovered nearly a century earlier.

McIntire called in Naval Hospital commanding officer Captain John Harper, his executive officer Captain Paul Duncan, and Washington internist Paul Dickens. The team surely concluded that the bleeding was somewhere in Franklin's lower gastrointestinal tract and, at the least, an emergency transfusion was needed. An infusion in the White House doctor's office raised his hemoglobin level to a slightly more reassuring 5.5.

The presidential calendar for May 5 has only one entry: Margaret "Daisy" Suckley, who had arrived by train from Poughkeepsie in time to dine with Franklin in his bedroom at 5:45 p.m. and stayed with him until 9:20 that evening. Their conversations at this nadir of Franklin's health is lost to history as Daisy destroyed her diary entry for that date. She had befriended him at the outset of his battle with polio, and the two had cultivated a close friendship since Franklin's years as Governor of New York. Daisy kept Franklin updated on the Dutchess County gossip he enjoyed hearing about. A devoted dog enthusiast, in November 1940 she had gifted him his famous Scotch terrier, Fala. It would be hard to find a woman to be more obsessed with or devoted to a man than Daisy was with her beloved "P." For Franklin, the arrangement worked perfectly.

Daisy's detailed diary, begun when Franklin assumed the presidency, broke off in July 1939 and did not resume with any regularity until March 1942—surprising, given the monumental intervening public and personal events: the campaign for a third term, and her gift to him of Fala, a world war. There are no entries about Franklin's reactions to Missy LeHand's devastating stroke, Sara Roosevelt's death, or Pearl Harbor. It seems odd for a dedicated diarist such as Daisy to omit so many important matters, especially since at other times she recorded even the most miniscule details of Franklin's life. But as Geoffrey C. Ward, the editor of the book that introduced the diary to the world notes, Daisy censored her material, having "destroy[ed] some of [her letters to FDR] and drastically edited others."[6]

Daisy appears to have bowdlerized her entries between late 1939 and early 1942 post facto, most likely because the medical problems she and Franklin never wanted revealed were so intrusive during this period as to have made them impossible to exclude. In subsequent entries, Daisy surmised that Franklin was experiencing "very bad trouble" with his blood in 1941, even if she misunderstood that "trouble's" precise nature. She wrote that Franklin had

---

6 Ward, G.C. ed., *Closest Companion, the Unknown Story of the Intimate Friendship between Franklin Roosevelt and Margaret Suckley.* Boston and New York: Houghton Mifflin, 1995.

"a lack of white corpuscles" as opposed to his well-documented loss of red blood cells. Her amateurish medical research found "only one disease" that matched what Daisy thought to be the problem, causing her to conclude that Franklin had leukemia—which, she noted fearfully, "is considered fatal over a period of time."[7] Franklin D. Roosevelt had a long list of illnesses, some of them potentially fatal, but leukemia wasn't one of them.

The effect of Daisy's censorship is compounded by the fact that she was also appointed by Franklin to be archivist of the presidential library he opened on June 30, 1941. Until 1963, she had oversight of his personal and family papers. It is fair to assume that nothing went into those archives—nor survived in her diary—that Daisy believed Franklin would not have wanted there, nor is it a stretch to assume that she assured him of this. Even when directly confronted about it, Daisy never admitted to keeping a diary. Its discovery, along with her correspondence from Franklin, found under her bed after her death at age 99 in 1991, was a complete surprise.

The morning of May 6, the day after Franklin's anemia was discovered, a bit of official business was too important to postpone. The "war cabinet" was convened in order to be updated about Harry Hopkins's recent meeting with Churchill in London.[8] At noon, Steve Early, with Ross McIntire in tow, called reporters together. Though the two men were well aware that Franklin had just undergone a life-saving emergency blood transfusion, Early told reporters, "Ross McIntire just came over to tell me that after the President finished his conference this morning with what you gentlemen call the 'war cabinet,' he saw the President and found that he has a degree and a half of temperature. Ross believes that he has eaten something that disagrees with him; he thinks he knows what it is and the situation will soon be cleared up; everything else is quite all right. The wisest thing to do this afternoon, is to keep him confined to his quarters."[9]

> McINTIRE: Slight gastrointestinal upset; we will have to give him a little time to straighten out.

> EARLY: So we are canceling his press conference.

---

7 *Suckley Diary.*

8 Secretary of State Cordell Hull, Treasury Secretary Henry Morgenthau, War Secretary Henry Stimson, Naval Secretary Frank Knox, Generals George Marshall and Henry "Hap" Arnold, Admiral Harold Stark, and Harry Hopkins.

9 Early's transcribed interactions with the press are found in scrapbooks he began keeping after Franklin assumed the presidency. The photos and press clippings contained in them are an extremely important research tool.

McINTIRE: It is nothing serious. I could not get Steve and I wanted to wait till he got back before we passed the word.

REPORTER: What did "Pa" [Watson] feed him?

EARLY: You will ruin "Pa" if you say anything like that.

McINTIRE: Off the record, for your information, we have a nice "stomach rolling" and we have to give it a few hours to get cleared up.

REPORTER: How did you stop him?

McINTIRE: He sent word over that he was not feeling so well.

A speech scheduled for May 10 to declare an "Unlimited National Emergency" in response to Nazi aggression was postponed. There was no sense of alarm in newspapers across the country, which reported nothing more than optimistic reports of a stomach ache and slight fever. Other than lunch with New York City Mayor Fiorello LaGuardia on May 7, a May 11 follow-up with Admiral Harold Stark of the war cabinet, and a brief visit by Robert Menzies, the prime minister of Australia, on May 12, Franklin did not leave his bedroom until May 13. He did interact with Missy and Harry Hopkins, both living in the White House at the time, and had sickroom visits from speechwriter Robert Sherwood, his son Elliott, and Princess Martha of Norway.

"The President has been ill all week and kept to his bed," Harold Ickes diarized on May 10. "According to Ross McIntire, it is an intestinal disturbance which is not particularly important but results in a temperature and leaves the President too weak to transact business. And so, no one has seen him, except of course the usual coterie, Harry and 'Missy,' etc." Cabinet members may have been in the dark about Franklin's illness but not Vincent Astor, who ended a May 15 letter to his friend, "I hope that you are feeling better now."[10]

"The President came down with an intestinal disturbance that seems to have caused a good deal of trouble," Ickes wrote on May 17. "The result has been that for ten days or two weeks he was in bed and practically no one could see him. Last Monday Ross McIntire told me that his temperature had gone down and that he was all right again, although still weak. Ross said positively, and 'Missy' confirmed it later, that the reason he had canceled his speech on Wednesday night was that he was not physically able

---

10 FDRL. The letter also briefly discusses Astor's espionage activity concerning the high-ranking Nazi, Rudolph Hess, as well as his use of *Nourmahal* to entertain South American dignitaries.

to make a speech. However during the week [Franklin] has been picking up and reports from people who have seen him are that he looks fine and acts again energetically. However, he did not get over to his office until Friday and the work undertaken has been light."

Laboratory reports from this crisis survived to be kept in the FDR Library among daughter Anna's files. The records reveal not just some of Franklin's medical aliases but also how his doctors approached the mysterious bleeding. They started out unsure of the source of blood loss—and apparently never found it. A complete gastrointestinal study with barium contrast was normal. No intestinal parasites were found. Test results for hemolysis (destruction of red cells), blood salt levels, and kidney functions were normal with the exception of a small amount of protein in Franklin's urine—a condition first noted a year earlier.

On May 15, Eleanor wrote to Anna, "I found Pa had really been quite ill & Dr. McIntire was worried because his red cells which should be up to 5,000,000 dropped suddenly to 2,800,000. He has had 2 transfusions & his tummy is cleared up and his color seems good, his blood is back to 4,000,000 ... no temperature for the last 4 days."[11] The fever likely was a reaction to transfusions. Press conferences for May 6, 9, and 13 were canceled due to "minor illness of the President." An additional transfusion on May 14 raised Franklin's hemoglobin level to 8.0, providing him enough energy to resume a limited schedule. Meeting with reporters on May 16, he began with an aside about his health. "Still feel a little weak, but otherwise I am coming along all right," he told the press. "Complexion is better, and everything else. It's a good thing." He then joked about Steve Early's absence in order to attend a golf tournament—and that was all there was to it.

On May 27, Franklin's first full day back at work, he delivered the postponed "Unlimited National Emergency" speech in a Fireside Chat at 9:30 p.m., then attended a reception and banquet at the White House for 210 guests followed by a midnight performance by composer Irving Berlin. Two days later, he left Washington for five days of rest in Hyde Park.

The intestinal bleeding recurred on June 12. A stool specimen revealed gross hemorrhage of red blood—six weeks after the problem first came to McIntire's attention. The next day's press conference was canceled due to an

---

11 Asbell, B., *Mother and Daughter, the Letters of Eleanor and Anna Roosevelt*. New York: Penguin, 1982, 131.

unspecified "minor illness" and Franklin did not return to work for another three days. On June 16, he confessed in a letter to Admiral William Leahy, then Ambassador to France, "I have written you very seldom because I have been more or less laid up with a low-grade infection, probably intestinal flu, since the first of May. The result is that my actual output of mail is about cut in half."[12] Medical records confirm that Franklin received at least eight transfusions in the three months after he was diagnosed.[13]

The list of possible explanations for a slow, undetected loss of eight pints of blood from the lower gastrointestinal tract over fourteen months includes toxic, immunological, vascular, structural, environmental, and parasitic causes. The blood in Franklin's stool was bright red. This excludes his stomach and upper small intestine as the source of leakage, because acid in those organs turns blood black—known to doctors as melena. Hemorrhoids—dilated veins in the rectal or anal region—large enough to leak that much would have alerted Franklin's medical aides long before May. Even if hemorrhoids were causing the bleeding, a minor surgical procedure would have relieved the condition. There is no evidence of a hemorrhoidectomy.

After years of research and consultations with scores of specialists, the best speculation is that Franklin's blood loss was caused by a condition that had not yet been described in the medical literature in 1941—radiation enteropathy—bowel damage from the radiotherapy used to treat his prostate cancer.[14] The time frame fits with the mystery medical procedure performed aboard *Tuscaloosa* in February 1940.

While McIntire and Early were trying to convince the American press that the President's illness was of little concern, Nazi spies arrived at a different conclusion. A top-secret message from an operative of the *Abwehr*, Hitler's espionage organization, reported to Berlin on June 19 that Franklin had "chronic uremia [kidney failure]" causing a "serious disturbance of consciousness as a result of constant application of a catheter in the urinary tract. Recurrent announcements indicating mild soreness of the throat and similar illnesses are made merely to camouflage his true condition." The agent attributed the information to one of the President's doctors, after the Nazi spy had "ingratiated

12 O'Brien, P.P., *The Second Most Powerful Man in the World*. Dutton, 2019, 159.
13 This statistic is gleaned from the laboratory reports in Anna's files, which reveal jumps in hemoglobin levels explicable only by transfusion.
14 https://www.mayoclinic.org/diseases-conditions/radiation-enteritis/symptoms-causes/syc-20355409.

himself to the capital's notoriously indiscreet 'high society' by posing as a scion of the noble Scottish clan of Douglas."[15,16]

McIntire reiterated the diagnosis of "mild intestinal influenza" to Walter Karig for a March 1942 article in a *Liberty*.[17] On March 22, 1951, he concocted another one for *U.S. News and World Report* in his characteristic "dumb like a fox" style.

"I would say that he didn't have a serious illness but we had one time that gave us a little concern. He developed a *mild* anemia [emphasis added]," McIntire told the magazine. "As I remember that was 1940. It was the day we went down to Staunton—he was doing something at the Woodrow Wilson place. I thought he didn't look too good and he didn't feel very well. He said, 'It's strange, I just don't feel very well—I feel that I've lost some pep,'" McIntire continued. "So when we got back to Washington we proceeded to get a blood picture, and sure enough, his blood had dropped down, so we immediately got busy to see what happened. This was over a short period—we found that he had an ordinary thing that lots of people have—he had a bleeding hemorrhoid that he hadn't noticed and blood had been dripping from this thing for quite a little time and brought him down some. But he picked up in no time flat—in fact no one ever noticed that—it was just that easy." Only the last ten words were true.

Missy LeHand had taken up residence at the governor's mansion in Albany and the White House so as to be available whenever Franklin needed her. By 1940 she required opiates to sleep.[18] The stress of the President's recent pro-longed illness taxed the limits of her endurance. On June 4, Missy was hostess of a formal White House dinner. As the evening stretched on with singing around the piano, she told Grace Tully she was not feeling well but refused to leave before Franklin did. Soon after he left, Missy screamed and collapsed— her heart had gone into an arrhythmia. Dr. McIntire and George Fox carried her upstairs to her apartment and sedated her.

Missy was bedridden at the White House for three weeks with pains in her chest, shoulder, and neck, requiring morphine and other sedatives to sleep. Franklin visited her several times. When a "sore throat" kept him away, he sent

15 Farago, L., *The Game of Foxes*. New York: David McKay Company, 1971, 330.
16 This description points to Franklin's loose-lipped urologist, William Calhoun Stirling.
17 Is The President Fit for a Third Term? *Liberty*, March 22, 1942.
18 Smith, K., 229.

a note signed, "Ever so much love, FDR."[19]After she developed a prolonged fever, Missy's doctors suspected a heart valve infection and hospitalized her. Thanks to sulfa antibiotics, the fever broke on June 27, but in the course of talking with a doctor, a blood clot broke off from her diseased valve, traveled to her brain, and blocked a major blood vessel.[20] The resultant stroke paralyzed Missy's right side and deprived her of the ability to speak.

Eleven top medical and surgical specialists, including cardiologists, neurosurgeons, gynecologists, urologists and psychiatrists, attended to her.[21] Franklin later wrote personal letters of thanks to all of them and paid for Missy's treatment. Despite the best medical care, including a long stay at Warm Springs for rehabilitation, Missy never recovered. Franklin amended his will to leave half the income from his estate to provide for her care. She died on July 31, 1944, while Franklin was aboard a Navy cruiser sailing from Hawaii to the Aleutian Islands. Eleanor attended the funeral mass in suburban Boston which was celebrated by soon-to be Archbishop of Boston, later Cardinal Richard J. Cushing.[22]

Franklin never changed his will after Missy's death. In January 1945, James asked why. "I owed her that much. She served me so well for so long and asked so little in return." His father responded.[23] To this day, the Roosevelt family pays to maintain her gravesite at Mount Auburn cemetery in Cambridge Massachusetts. Grace Tully assumed Missy's secretarial duties and Anna moved into the White House to assist her father in December 1943, but no one could ever come close to replacing Missy LeHand as Franklin's most intimate confidante, adviser, and companion.

---

19 *Ibid.*, 241.
20 Specifically, the middle cerebral artery of her dominant left cerebral hemisphere.
21 The list of "thank you" letters from Franklin can be found at PPF 3737, FDRL. One of the neurosurgeons, Dr. James W. Watts, went on to perform a disastrous pre-frontal lobotomy on Joseph Kennedy's daughter, Rosemary. Another was Frederick A. Reuter, Professor of Clinical Urology at George Washington School of Medicine. A detailed letter of Dr. Reuter to Ross McIntire outlining the treatment for protein in the urine of "John Cash", allegedly the son of a White House policeman, is in the McIntire Files of the FDRL. Probably not by coincidence, the name appears on the list of Franklin's aliases and Franklin had had the problem since 1940. The list also includes radiologist Charles F. Behrens, who interpreted most of Franklin's x-rays and also likely supervised his radiation therapy.
22 Cushing celebrated the same rites for John F. Kennedy in November 1963.
23 Smith, K., 269.

On June 5, the day after Missy took ill, Lucy Mercer, now Mrs. Winthrop Rutherfurd, came to the White House, listed in the official log as "Mrs. Paul Johnson." The purpose of her two-hour visit was ostensibly to ask Franklin's help to get her ailing husband admitted to Walter Reed Hospital. After her apparent breakup with Franklin in 1918, Lucy married Rutherfurd, a widower thirty years her senior. She assumed the care of his children and had a child by him, Barbara, who Franklin referred to as his godchild. Over the years, Franklin and Lucy exchanged letters and phone calls and, in later years met secretly for an unknown number of times in Washington's Rock Creek Park. The White House operator was instructed to put Lucy's calls through to the president, who spoke with her in French to foil eavesdropping. Lucy attended all four of Franklin's inaugurations, the first three courtesy of tickets sent by Missy LeHand.[24]

A majority of Americans sympathized with Britain over Nazi Germany but opposed sending troops to fight overseas. On June 22, Hitler launched Operation Barbarossa, a full-scale invasion of the U.S.S.R. In the Pacific, the Japanese were moving into French-held Indochina—today's Vietnam, Cambodia, and Laos—and threatening British and Dutch colonies in Southeast Asia.

Franklin wanted a face-to-face meeting with Churchill, but German submarines made trans-Atlantic voyages too hazardous. An ultra-secret rendezvous aboard naval vessels was arranged off the southwest coast of Newfoundland at Placentia Bay.[25] Neither Eleanor nor Secretary of State Hull were given advance notice. "Even at my ripe old age," Franklin wrote Daisy Suckley. "I feel a thrill in making a get-away—especially from the American press." [26,27]

On August 3, Franklin left Washington for New London, Connecticut, to board the presidential yacht *Potomac*, ostensibly for a fishing trip off Cape Cod.[28] The cloak-and-dagger aspects began on August 5, when he transferred

---

24 Persico, J., *Roosevelt's Secret War.* New York: Random House, 2002, 227.

25 The meeting was held near Argentia, a village where a military base had been granted by Britain to America as part of a "Destroyers for Bases Agreement" reached on August 30, 1940.

26 One of Franklin's favorite pastimes was reading murder mysteries. He even developed a plot of his own, submitted it for enhancement by six well-known authors and had it published in *Liberty* magazine in 1935. "The President's Murder Mystery" was made into a movie starring Betty Furness in 1936.

27 Ward, *Closest Companion*, 140.

28 The afternoon before he had spent three hours at the White House with "Mrs. Paul

to cruiser USS *Augusta*—leaving his presidential flag flying on *Potomac* to indicate he was still aboard. He arrived at Placentia Bay on August 9 with an entourage that included the now indispensable Ross McIntire.[29] Churchill had made his Atlantic crossing aboard battleship HMS *Prince of Wales*.

"I like him & lunching alone broke the ice both ways,"[30] Franklin wrote Daisy. During the eight-day conference, Franklin and Winston drafted the Atlantic Charter, an early vision of what would result in the founding of the United Nations. The charter pledged that "all men in all lands may live out their lives in freedom from fear and from want."

Soon after returning to Washington, Franklin received word that Sara, now 87, had taken ill. He found her on her deathbed at Springwood and reminisced with her for the remainder of the day. After a brief rally, Sara went into a coma and died with Franklin at her side. As if on cue, a large oak nearby came crashing to the ground, even though there had been no wind nor rain. Sara was laid to rest in the cemetery of St. James Episcopal Church next to Mr. James.

On December 13, 1941, an article entitled "Is the President a Well Man Today?" appeared in *Liberty*. Author Walter Karig admitted that when Americans saw the president in newsreels, they left movie theaters "shaking their heads and saying, 'The President does not look well at all.'" Steve Early and Marvin McIntyre, both veterans of the movie newsreel industry, gave an excuse that audiences were used to seeing professional actors whose features were enhanced by professional makeup artists. Franklin, in contrast "goes barefaced ... without a dab of powder on his chin ... His face is rugged, with strong contours that throw shadows [so that] he'll always look twenty years older in the movies." Franklin had probably been using makeup to camouflage his melanoma for years.[31]

The remainder of the article was devoted to convincing readers that Franklin was in tip-top shape. Ross McIntire claimed that Franklin's health was better than it had been a year ago. "Heart? Steady as a chronometer. Lungs? Like a long-distance swimmer's." Perhaps there was "a little trouble" with

Johnson,"—Lucy Mercer Rutherfurd.
29 By this time, Franklin required twice-a-day treatment and could not be away from the only doctor who could provide it in secrecy. McIntire's whereabouts are difficult to trace, though he was not in Warm Springs when Franklin died.
30 Ward, *Closest Companion*, 141.
31 Pancake makeup was invented by Max Factor & Co. in the late 1930s for use in color movies.

the president's digestion last spring due to a "low-grade intestinal infection" that required a diet of pureed spinach and strained mashed string beans and cereal. The president had lost ten pounds, and was now permitted a daily meal of steak, said McIntire. There was, of course, no mention of blood loss. Two photographs accompanied the article. The first showed Franklin in a somber pose as he had looked eight years earlier, an apparently less healthy man than a recent image taken while he was smiling and looking vigorous—the melanoma above his left eyebrow nowhere to be seen.

Shielding Franklin's disability was far more successful than the president and members of his innermost circle could possibly have imagined. Even White House staff marveled at the difference between perception and reality. "The door opened and the Secret Service guard wheeled in the President of the United States. Startled, I looked down at him," J.B. West recalled of his second day as chief usher at the White House in 1941. "It was only then that I realized that Franklin D. Roosevelt was totally paralyzed. Immediately I understood why the fact had been kept so secret. Everybody knew that the president had been stricken with infantile paralysis and his recovery was legend, but few people were aware how completely the disease had handicapped him."[32]

Franklin received word of the attack on Pearl Harbor by telephone from Secretary of the Navy, Frank Knox, at 1:47 p.m. on Sunday, December 7. Grace Tully recalled he appeared calm as reports throughout the afternoon disclosed the full extent of damage the Japanese had inflicted. "With each new message he shook his head grimly and tightened the expression of his mouth," Tully observed. Nineteen warships had been sunk or damaged. Battleship *Arizona* rested on the harbor bottom, along with nearly 1,100 of its crewmen. More than 300 warplanes had been damaged or destroyed, most of them on the ground. American casualties numbered 2,403 dead and 1,178 wounded while just 29 Japanese aircraft were shot down—the most lopsided defeat in American military history.

On December 8, Franklin addressed a joint session of Congress, famously labeling the attack on December 7 "a date which will live in infamy." The next evening Americans gathered around their radios to hear the now familiar voice reassure them: "We will gain the inevitable triumph—so help us God." Hitler declared war on the United States on December 11, sparing criticism

---

32 West, J.B., *Upstairs at the White House*. New York: Coward, McCann & Geoghegan, 1973, 17.

of Franklin by Charles Lindbergh and his Nazi-sympathizing followers about starting a two-front war.

Vincent Astor had emerged from the Great War with an interest in intelligence gathering. In 1927, he organized a cadre of powerful gentry who shared a common interest in espionage, national defense, and a robust New York City economy into a secret fraternity he called "The Room."[33] The group met monthly in a nondescript apartment at 34 East 62nd Street in Manhattan to discuss global politics as well as social, military, and economic matters. The roster was an aristocracy of wealth and power—spymaster David K. E. Bruce, the son-in-law of treasury secretary Andrew Mellon;[34] chairman of U.S. Steel J.P. Morgan Jr., and Winthrop W. Aldrich, President of Chase Manhattan Bank, to mention a few; as well as high-ranking British military officers, TR's son Kermit, influential legal professionals, scientists, athletes and publishers.[35]

After Franklin assumed the presidency, Astor was his personal spymaster. This aspect of their relationship is worthy of a book of its own, but beyond the scope of this work.[36,37,38,39]

One of Vincent Astor's boldest acts of counterespionage was particularly effective at the outset of World War II. In 1941, the Diesel Research Company, a front created by Nazi intelligence, rented an office in his *Newsweek* Building

33 Two sources stand out as the best information about "The Room." Dorwart, J.M., "The Roosevelt-Astor Espionage Ring." *New York History* July 1981;63(3): 307–322 and Villano, W., "Vincent Astor. Millionaire, Philanthropist, Spy and Friend of President Roosevelt." https://artsandculture.google.com/story/vincent-astor-u-s-national-archives/EgVxQyhXXB8A8A?hl=en (last accessed April 17, 2023).

34 Bruce was an outstanding career diplomat and became OSS chief in Europe from 1943 to 1945, with the rank of colonel. He was America's chief spymaster during World War II.

35 Astor sought out guest lecturers such as William J. "Wild Bill" Donovan, America's most decorated soldier during the war, and playwright, best-selling novelist, and former British intelligence officer, W. Somerset Maugham.

36 By far the best reference about the Astor/FDR relationship is a monograph by William Villano, published during his tenure at the FDR Library. https://artsandculture.google.com/exhibit/vincent-astor-u-s-national-archives/wQ2hXHF9?

37 Villano, W., "Socialite and Spy Master: Vincent Astor, FDR's Area Controller of Intelligence for New York." *Bulletin of the Franklin D. Roosevelt Presidential Library and Museum* November 16, 2016. https://fdr.blogs.archives.gov/2016/11/16/socialite-and-spy-master-vincent-astor-fdrs-area-controller-of-intelligence-for-new-york/.

38 Dorwart, J.M., "The Roosevelt-Astor Espionage Ring." *New York History,* Quarterly Journal of the New York State Historical Association, July 1981;LXII(3):307–322.

39 Astor's letters to FDR about this espionage are in the Grace Tully papers, FDRL.

in New York City.[40] Adjacent offices were provided to the FBI. Hidden microphones and cameras were installed. With the cooperation of a double agent, 33 spies were arrested, including Fritz Duquesne, the chief *Abwehr's* operative in North America. Nineteen pleaded guilty and the others went to trial. On January 2, 1942, the defendants were collectively sentenced to over 300 years in prison. Nazi espionage in America was devastated.[41]

---

40 The building was located at 444 Madison Avenue.
41 https://www.fbi.gov/history/famous-cases/duquesne-spy-ring.

■ Chapter 19
■ Dr. Win the War

On December 22, 1941, Winston Churchill and his senior military staff arrived in Washington for Arcadia, a three-week conference to coordinate military operations and codify a "Germany first" strategy.[1] Churchill took up residence in the White House Blue Room. One morning, eager to tell his visitor the name he'd thought of for his world peace organization, Franklin wheeled himself into Churchill's quarters and caught him coming out of the bath—stark naked. "The Prime Minister of Great Britain has nothing to conceal from the President of the United States," Churchill exclaimed.[2] "He's pink and white all over," Franklin told Grace Tully.[3]

"Old Doctor Roosevelt" became "Dr. Win the War." "You know I am a juggler, and I never let my right hand know what my left hand does,"[4] Franklin bragged to his friend and neighbor, Treasury Secretary "Henry the Morgue" Morgenthau Jr. "I may have one policy for Europe and one diametrically opposite for North and South America. I may be entirely inconsistent, and furthermore I am perfectly willing to mislead and tell untruths if it will help win the war."[5]

By March, the Japanese were driving outnumbered and undersupplied American forces from the Philippines and seizing smaller Pacific islands in a push toward Hawaii. Franklin sensed a bold move was needed to bolster American spirits. On April 18, sixteen B-25 bombers led by General James H. Doolittle took off from aircraft carrier *Hornet* and bombed Tokyo and other targets on Honshu, the main island of the Japanese archipelago. The planes continued westward until they ran out of fuel over China and the Soviet Union. The damage inflicted was negligible but succeeded in what it was intended to do. When asked where the planes had come from, Franklin

---

1 https://en.wikipedia.org/wiki/Arcadia_Conference.
2 Sherwood, 442.
3 Tully, G., *Franklin Delano Roosevelt—My Boss*. Chicago: Peoples Book Club, 1949, 305.
4 Franklin learned this advice from the New Testament, Matthew 6:3.
5 Roosevelt, quoting himself, speaking to a special study group on Latin America; memorandum of a conversation between Roosevelt and Morgenthau, May 15, 1942, *Presidential Diary*, p. 1093, Henry Morgenthau Jr. papers, Franklin D. Roosevelt Library, Hyde Park, New York.

answered "Shangri-la," a reference to the mythical Himalayan utopia made famous by James Hilton's popular 1933 novel, *Lost Horizon*, and a 1937 film based on the book.

In June, the Japanese and American fleets squared off near Midway Island. The Americans had broken the Japanese code and knew their plans. Four Japanese aircraft carriers were sunk. One American carrier was lost. The battle of Midway was the turning point of the Pacific war and enabled the "Germany first" strategy.[6]

News on the other side of the world was grim. Axis troops controlled most of Europe and North Africa. Stalin's armies were sustaining huge losses. Top American military commanders pushed for an immediate attack on northern Europe but Franklin sided with Churchill against it. Instead, the Allies launched Operation Torch, an invasion of North Africa. American forces went ashore in Morocco and Algeria on November 7.[7]

On January 14, 1943, Franklin flew to Casablanca, Morocco, to confer with Churchill. Wartime precautions mandated a cruising altitude no lower than 13,000 feet, but Dr. McIntire lowered the ceiling to 9,000 out of concern for "the President's bad heart." Even so, Harry Hopkins noted Franklin looked pale.

At Churchill's insistence, Franklin continued to defer a cross-channel invasion of France—this time targeting southern Europe through Sicily. Also at Casablanca, Franklin announced the Allies would accept nothing less than unconditional surrender. Churchill's penchant for talking and drinking well into the night taxed Franklin's endurance. He wrote Daisy about "a bit of bronchial trouble & a slight temperature."[8]

After returning stateside on January 31, Franklin found it difficult to stay healthy, writing to Churchill about a "strange African bug," "Gambia fever" as he told Eleanor, that put him to bed for days and left him exhausted.[9] "It

---

6 https://www.armyheritage.org/wp-content/uploads/2020/06/Europe_First_US_Army_ Heritage_Final_Edit.pdf.

7 Churchill's opposition stemmed from the repercussions of his disastrous decision at Gallipoli as First Lord of the Admiralty during World War I and the depleted state of the British military following Dunkirk and the Battle of Britain. This topic has been well-addressed in dozens of Churchill biographies, both positive and negative.

8 Ward, *Closest Companion*, 200.

9 Roosevelt and Brough, *A Rendezvous With Destiny: The Roosevelts of Hyde Park.* London:

is the P's fourth day in bed, & he still feels somewhat miserable though his fever has gone," Daisy wrote. "Last Tuesday, without any warning, he fell ill at about noon. He lay on his study sofa & slept 'til 4:30, when he found he had a temp. of 102. The Dr. found it was a toxic poisoning, but they can't ascribe it to anything they know of ... On Wednesday they gave him 4 doses of a sulpha drug—from which he will have to recover."

Franklin was still sick after ten days. Daisy quoted him as saying he "feels like a rag & is much annoyed at himself."[10] She also noticed for the first time "his hand sometimes shakes."[11]

By this time, surgery and makeup had cosmetically erased the dark mole above Franklin's left eye. Comparison photos published on the tenth anniversary of his presidency didn't raise any eyebrows (pun intended).[12]

Boston surgeon Frank H. Lahey had been appointed by Ross McIntire to lead the Navy's Procurement and Assignment Service in November 1941. The group was responsible for recruiting and placing medical personnel and was comprised of a multispecialty medical brain trust that included at least three doctors who would later treat Franklin: Chairman Lahey, Washington urologist William Calhoun "Pete" Stirling, Jr., and Atlanta internist James T. Paullin.[13]

Franklin's prostate cancer became an issue during the winter of 1942–1943. New forms of treatment had been discovered since he had been diagnosed. In 1941, Canadian-American physician Charles Huggins made a groundbreaking discovery—reducing or opposing the effect of male hormones (testosterone) could reverse the spread of the disease.[14] This was the

---

W.H Allen 1977, 334.

10 *Ibid.*, March 9, 1943.

11 *Ibid.*

12 AP Wirephoto, January 13, 1943.

13 Paullin and Lahey became part of McIntire's "honorary board of consultants" who were called in to evaluate Franklin in late March, 1944. Both men became primary figures in the cover-up of his medical problems.

14 "Prostatic cancer is influenced by androgenic (male hormone) activity in the body. At least with respect to serum phosphatases [a recently discovered enzyme detectible in the blood], wide-spread cancer of the prostate cancer is inhibited by eliminating androgens [male hormones] through castration or neutralization of their activity by estrogen [female hormone] injection." Huggins, C., Hodges, C.V., "Studies on Prostatic Cancer: I. The Effect of Castration, of Estrogen, and of Androgen Injection on Serum Phosphatases in Metastatic Carcinoma of the Prostate." *Cancer Research* 1941;1:293–297. Huggins was

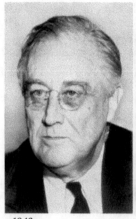
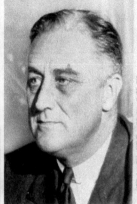

1943   1933

first demonstration that cancer could be controlled by chemicals—making it possible to treat prostate cancer with orchiectomy [removal of the testicles], the body's principal source of the hormone. Urologist William Calhoun Stirling, Stephen Early's regular bridge and golf partner,[15] evaluated the president and recommended an unspecified surgical procedure.[16] Orchiectomy is high on the list of possibilities. According to Walter Trohan, Stirling was reluctant to take on such a prominent patient alone and asked Dr. Lahey to evaluate the case, who allegedly concurred with the need for an operation. Franklin declined, citing his busy wartime schedule.[17] Later in 1943, Lahey concluded the cancer had progressed to the point where surgery was no longer an option.[18] While no evidence exists, it is logical to assume Franklin was treated with hormonal therapy. Contrary to the myth later created by his daughter, Franklin *always* had access to the most cutting-edge medical care.

---

awarded the Nobel Prize for Medicine in 1966.

15 Personal communication with Margheritta Allardice.

16 Stirling's professional involvement with Franklin was confirmed by his daughter, Margheritta Allardice. Mrs. Allardice had been working in her father's Washington office and had vivid memories of her father's involvement with the President. They became estranged in August 1943 over her father's objection to her marrying a Jew. They briefly reconnected shortly before Stirling's death when he wanted to meet his grandchildren (personal communication between Margheritta "Mickey" Allardice and the author).

17 Trohan, *Political Animals*, 198.

18 *Ibid*. The reason for not performing surgery is unknown, but the presence of bone metastases is a possibility.

In late September, Daisy wrote that Franklin had a "pain in his side," the first hint cancer might have begun to cause abdominal problems. Daisy implored him to discuss it with McIntire, but the patient shook off any concern. "The pain had moved & the doctor had left," she confided to her diary.[19] On September 29, Franklin was lethargic and "a little worried about swelling in the ankles when he is tired." Peripheral edema (swelling of the legs) is often a sign of poor circulation or heart failure.

On October 18, Daisy wrote that Franklin "fell asleep twice while trying to write a message to Congress ... He is just *too* tired, *too* often. I can't help worrying about him."[20] On October 20, Franklin informed Daisy he had "the grippe," ached all over,[21] and had a fever up to 104 and ¼. Ten days later he was still feeling "very tired" and "rather miserable."

Daisy wrote on November 5, "The P. was very tired after his long day—he was keyed up and couldn't relax. He has started taking coffee for breakfast again, as, on the long trip [to Tehran], there won't be anything else to drink. It is obviously not good for him; it shows in his hands which become nervous & a little shaky."

Franklin was scheduled to leave for a summit meeting in Tehran on Armistice Day, November 11, 1943. That afternoon Dr. Lahey visited the White House, supposedly on official business. But he had likely come for a different reason. Years later, medical sleuth Dr. Harry Goldsmith found a newsletter published by an exclusive New Hampshire country club, of which Lahey was a member.[22] The document revealed details of a conversation between Franklin and Lahey concerning the conditions by which the doctor would accept the position of his consulting surgeon:

Lahey would accept no "undue remuneration."

He would not be made an admiral or a general.

He had never voted for FDR and didn't plan to in 1944.

---

19 *Suckley diary*, September 30, 1943.
20 Grace Tully later described "nodding off " or "dozing" over his work a few months later, raising the possibility these episodes were something quite different than fatigue.
21 Grace Tully later described "nodding off " or "dozing" over his work a few months later, raising the possibility these episodes were something quite different than fatigue.
22 Lahey's membership was confirmed by the Club Manager in a conversation with the author on November 14, 2021.

He considered Franklin the most important person in the world, making his health of great concern to Lahey.

"Do you still want me as your consulting surgeon?" Lahey asked the president. Franklin laughed and replied. "Thank you for your frankness, I will send my plane for you every Monday morning."[23]

Also appearing on the White House calendar on that day was Dr. John W. Norcross, an internist and chief of medicine at Lahey's clinic. When he was later confronted by Dr. Harry Goldsmith about the visit, Norcross was caught off guard and initially "forgot" he had met the president.[24]

On the evening of November 11, Franklin began his journey to Tehran, boarding the newly commissioned battleship USS *Iowa* at Newport News, Virginia, accompanied by Ross McIntire and Harry Hopkins. They were joined there by high-ranking military officers and arrived at Oran, Algeria, on November 20. He was met there by Elliott, Franklin Jr. and General Dwight D. Eisenhower and that evening took a three-hour flight to Tunisia. The next evening, he flew to Cairo to join Churchill and Chinese Nationalist leader Chiang Kai-shek for five days of meetings. FDR and Churchill went on to Tehran on November 27, where Stalin was waiting. "Churchill suffered an episode of chest pain while staying at the White House and without benefit of ECG or a second opinion, his physician, Lord Moran, was of the opinion that Churchill had suffered a 'heart attack.'"[25] Out of concern for Franklin's heart, McIntire once again insisted the plane fly below cloud cover. When Elliott asked why, the doctor brusquely replied, "Nothing over 7,500—that's tops."[26]

For security concerns,[27] Franklin relocated to Stalin's quarters at the Russian embassy and hosted a banquet where the "Big Three" discussed plans for the war. At that dinner, "Roosevelt was about to say something when suddenly, in the flick of an eye, he turned green and great drops of sweat began to bead off his face; he put a shaky hand to his forehead," interpreter and later ambassador

23 Undated newsletter of the Bald Peak Colony Club, Lake Winnipesaukee, New Hampshire. Goldsmith, Harry L. *Conspiracy of Silence* Bloomington IN: IUniverse, 2007, 119.
24 Goldsmith, H.L., *Conspiracy of Silence*, Bloomington IN: iUniverse, 2007, 175.
25 Allister Vale, J., Scadding, J.W., "Did Winston Churchill Suffer a Myocardial Infarction in the White House at Christmas 1941?" *Journal of the Royal Society of Medicine* 2017;110(12):483–492.
26 Crispell, K.R., Gomez, C.F., *Hidden Illness in the White House.* Durham, NC: Duke University Press, 1988, 76.
27 Roosevelt and Brough, *RWD*, 351.

to the Soviet Union Charles Bohlen recalled.[28] "We were all caught by surprise. The president made no complaint, and none of us detected any sign of discomfort. Hopkins had the President wheeled to his room, where the White House doctor … made a quick examination and, to the relief of everybody, reported nothing more than a mild attack of indigestion." The President retired for the evening. The next morning, Hopkins told Bohlen he had been quite concerned—as had Bohlen—until they heard McIntire's diagnosis.[29]

Franklin appeared to have recovered the next day, but the mysterious episode had led to speculation about the cause. Historian Robert H. Ferrell dismissed the idea that Franklin might have been poisoned, as was rumored at the time, stating, "It seemed more natural, more likely, to define the attack as a sign of stomach cancer."[30] Ferrell's impression is given credence by at least three other attacks of severe abdominal pain Franklin experienced in 1944.

When a member of the British delegation asked Churchill whether Franklin had said much during that day's meeting with Stalin, the prime minister replied, "Harry Hopkins said that the president was inept. He was asked a lot of questions and gave the wrong answers."[31] Nonetheless, the primary consequence of the summit, pushed through over Churchill's continuing objection, was to give Stalin his long-awaited second front by proceeding with Operation Overlord, a cross-channel invasion of France planned for the spring of 1944. An agreement was also made about Poland's postwar borders.

Upon Franklin's return stateside on December 17, Dr. Lahey sent his patient a carefully worded letter "I hope that you have recovered from your cold," he wrote, "and while this may represent Hibernian [Irish] sentiment, I would like to express to you my admiration for what you have recently accomplished and for your capacity to take the physical handicaps which I knew went with it."[32]

Shortly before Christmas 1943, Franklin's daughter Anna came to Washington from her home in Seattle.[33] "With no preliminary talks or discussions I found

---

28 Bohlen was appointed Ambassador to the Soviet Union by Dwight Eisenhower in April 1953.
29 Bohlen, C.E., *Witness to History: 1929–1969*. New York: W.W. Norton, 1973, 143–144.
30 Ferrell, R.H., *The Dying President*. Columbia, MO: University of Missouri Press, 1988, 17.
31 Wilson Moran, C.M., *Churchill: Taken from the Diaries of Lord Moran*. London: Constable, 1966, 150, quoted in Burns, J.M., *Roosevelt: Soldier of Freedom*, 409.
32 *Ibid.*, 120.
33 Anna's first appearance in FDR's calendar was on December 20, identified as "Mrs. John Boettinger."

myself trying to take over little chores that I felt would relieve Father of some of the pressure under which he was constantly working. After a couple of weeks I asked Father if he'd mind if I resigned my job on the newspaper and stayed on to help him," Anna recalled.[34] "It was immaterial to me whether my job was helping to plan the 1944 campaign, pouring tea for General De Gaulle or filling father's empty cigarette case. All that mattered was relieving a greatly overburdened man of a few details of work and to make his life as pleasant as possible when a few moments opened up for relaxation."[35] Anna assumed the roles of social hostess and gatekeeper previously held by Missy LeHand. There was one constraint—her father insisted she must not keep a diary.

About this time, a number of Franklin's close associates began to see signs of physical decline. "The President developed some sort of bronchial affliction in Tehran, which gave him a wracking cough. It took him a long time to shake it off," Sam Rosenman wrote. "While Tehran was a high point in the President's career as Commander-in-Chief of our armed forces and as our leader in foreign affairs, it seemed to me to be also the turning point of his physical career ... although at that time we did not see it." Rosenman's observation is accurate, but his accounts of later events appear to be intentionally incomplete. He had been a member of Franklin's innermost circle of advisers since his gubernatorial days and was privy to the deepest secrets of his boss's health.

"It is elementary that any man in his sixties is unlikely to have the same resiliency and capacity for absorption of work as one in his fifties, or his forties, or younger," Grace Tully wrote. "The Boss not only grew older in the manner of all human beings but he also faced responsibilities that intensified with the years, and he had no opportunity for genuine relaxation from those responsibilities. His so-called vacations were punctuated by periods of daily work dropped on his desk, wherever it was, by air-borne mail pouches or a car filled with radio and telegraph equipment. So it was that in the later years I observed the signs of cumulative weariness, the dark circles that never quite faded from under his eyes, the more pronounced shake in his hand as he lit his cigarette, the easy slump that developed in his shoulders as he sat at a desk that was always covered with work."[36,37] Tully's observations are an important

---

34 The Seattle *Post-Intelligencer* was published by her husband John Boettinger, who was in the military, stationed in Europe. Anna was editor of the women's pages.
35 Asbell, *Mother and Daughter*, 175.
36 Tully, 273–274.
37 Tully was also the first to mention the presence of "Mrs. Rutherford" [sic] at Warm Springs in April, 1945, but the potentially bombshell revelation went largely unnoticed.

historical record, but her explanation for his behavior, like those offered by many others, was naïve.

■ Chapter 20
■ Never-Ending Exhaustion

On Christmas Eve 1943, Franklin gave a Fireside Chat during a three-day weekend visit to Hyde Park. A few coughs can be heard on the recording, but his voice is clear and resonant. The next evening, the FDR Library was the setting for a party honoring the soldiers of the 240th M.P. Battalion stationed at Hyde Park. Enlisted man Garrett C. Wilcox, no fan of the president, kept a cynically entertaining diary.[1] His firsthand observations of Franklin's health are in stark contrast to the picture being painted for the American public. Wilcox identified himself by his service number and sarcastically employed reverential capitalization.

"At about eight in the evening an old man was wheeled in by his wife. His hair was sparse and iron grey. Face red-blotched and hand so shaky that He had the need of holding fast to the arms of his wheelchair. To watch Him intently, as did 32916555, was to expect a paralyzing stroke at any moment. The soldier had seen several members of his own family die shortly after a series of strokes, and His present appearance was all too familiar. So much had been said about His powerful and charming voice that a display of personal magnetism was to be expected. Eleanor urged Him to talk, but cautioned the assembly that He couldn't be expected to speak for long. A weak, toneless voice came forth, several times rising in pleasant modulations, but always sinking again in the manner of a man barely able to keep himself alive. He spoke of Tehran and the issues there and decisions arrived at with Marshall [sic] Stalin and Premier Churchill; this was all fresh in His mind, as He had only just returned from Iran. He had been favorably impressed with Marshall [sic] Stalin but the question naturally arose in the mind of one soldier whether He would have perceived a knife behind the smile of the Marshall [sic], assuming there was one. St. Franklin spoke on for perhaps twenty minutes, guided and managed at all times by Eleanor."[2] There was no mention of illness on December 21 and 28 press conferences. Daisy Suckley's diary describes Franklin feeling "a little miserably" on December 28. On December 29, the presidential schedule

---

1 The author located Wilcox's son by phone, living in New York City. He insisted his father was a lifelong Democrat.
2 Wilcox Diary, *Westbrook Pegler Papers*, Herbert Hoover Library, North Branch, Iowa.

came to an abrupt halt until January 6. "Day by Day" reports the illness as a "cold."

The "cold" forced postponement of the State of the Union address. It was eventually given as a Fireside Chat on January 11, 1944, and began with an excuse. "It has been my custom to deliver these annual messages in person, and they have been broadcast to the nation," Franklin explained over the radio. "I intended to follow this same custom this year. But, like a great many other people, I have had the flu and although I am practically recovered, my doctor simply would not let me."[3,4] A recently discovered film, withheld from distribution at the time, reveals a haggard president delivering an excerpt from the speech, notably his extraordinary "second bill of rights."[5]

There is vague evidence that Franklin had experienced something far more serious than the flu. With *Chicago Tribune* reporter Walter Trohan as his source, Dr. Karl Wold reported in *Look* magazine in 1949, "About this time a parade of doctors was called to the White House. Everyone refused to talk. But some of the physicians privately discussed Roosevelt's symptoms. They agreed that he had a stroke and was suffering from general deterioration and two of them doubted he could live until July 1, 1944."[6] Wold's claims are uncorroborated, but it would not be unreasonable to postulate that a small intracranial hemorrhage occurred at this time that triggered Franklin's seizures.[7]

On January 18, Franklin's first press conference after his three-week illness began with humor. "I want to assure you that I am no longer contagious and Dr. McIntire hopes that none of you are contagious," Franklin wisecracked, getting a laugh. But the "flu" was nowhere near as mild as he was suggesting, nor was he even close to having recovered. Even the perpetual Pollyanna Ross McIntire wrote Franklin had returned from Tehran with a severe pulmonary condition that left him bedridden for over a week with coughing spells that produced "thick, tenacious mucus." For three months, said McIntire, this condition "racked him by day and broke his rest at night" but "more disturbing

---

3 Roosevelt, F., "Fireside Chat Number 28, State of the Union Address," January 11, 1944. http://FDRLibrary.marist.edu FDRLibrary.marist.edu or FDRL.org.

4 *Ibid.*

5 Producer Michael Moore discovered the film at a North Carolina library and used it in his 2007 film, *Sicko.*

6 Wold, K.C., "The Truth About FDR's Health." *Look*, February 15, 1949.

7 Stroke from Intracranial hemorrhage is far more likely to cause subsequent seizures than one from a blood vessel occlusion.

than anything else ... there was the definite loss of his usual ability to come back quickly."[8]

On February 2, Franklin went to Bethesda Naval Hospital for treatment of his heart disease—in the guise of undergoing minor surgery. The cover story was that for twenty years he'd had a wen, a benign wartlike growth, growing on the back of his head, which was now causing discomfort when his hat rubbed against it and he'd decided to have it removed. Anna and Daisy were invited to ride with him to the hospital. "I think it will be more of an operation than they imply, but I hope not," Daisy confided to her diary. "Four doctors are to be there—even a *wen*, if on a P. of the U.S., is an important matter!"[9]

The truth was not disclosed until December 4, 1979, when the operating surgeon, chief of plastic surgery Dr. George Webster, gave his recollections of the event in a letter to Dr. Harry Goldsmith.[10] Webster told Goldsmith that he had not had a chance to examine the president before his arrival at the hospital but had been told by Admiral McIntire that the wen was "about the size of a hen's egg and almost exactly in the midline where the hat band would hit the head." That description proved accurate. No fewer than seven doctors were in the operating room.[11]

The optimal positioning to minimize bleeding for a patient undergoing this operation would have been lying face down, but Franklin and his doctors had been avoiding that posture, which caused him to become short of breath. He had even resorted to sleeping with his upper body propped up on pillows. Known in medial parlance as orthopnea, this phenomenon is caused by failure of the heart's left ventricle. "The President could not very well lie down for this procedure," Webster wrote. Instead, Franklin was seated in his wheelchair, his head supported by a device fashioned by the

---

8 McIntire, 182; *U.S. News & World Report,* March 22, 1951.

9 *Suckley Diary,* February 2, 1944.

10 Dr. George Webster to Dr. Harry Goldsmith, December 4, 1979, quoted in Goldsmith, *A Conspiracy of Silence,* 51.

11 The list includes McIntire; the hospital's two top officials, Captain John Harper, the chief of staff, and his executive officer, Captain Paul Duncan; a cardiologist [unnamed but most probably Howard Bruenn]; Captain Louis Gilje, the chief of general surgery; Captain Winchell McKendree Craig, the chief of neurosurgery, a position he'd held at the Mayo Clinic until joining the navy; anesthesiologist Captain John W. Pender, Craig's colleague from Mayo, and Captain George Webster, chief of plastic surgery, who performed the operation.

hospital's chief neurosurgeon, Dr. Winchell "Wink" McKendree Craig.[12] Local anesthesia was used. Daisy and Anna were asked if they would like to witness the procedure but declined, and luckily so, since the operation was complicated when a hemorrhage from the operative wound soaked Franklin's undershirt in blood.[13] The hospital's pathologist diagnosed a tissue sample as a "benign epidermoid cyst."[14]

Webster's letter told of a problem far more significant than a wen. "The removal of the epidermoid cyst was an incidental part of the hospital visit for which he came out from the White House for x-rays to see about his 'cigarette cough,'" Webster wrote. "On x-ray he was found to have some pulmonary edema [fluid in the lungs] and was, in effect, in early mild cardiac failure. This was recognized and he was immediately digitalized [given the drug digitalis]. Admiral McIntire had called Dr. Howard Bruenn, a naval reserve officer and cardiologist who was a good friend of mine from my days at Columbia-Presbyterian Medical Center in New York City where he was an attending cardiologist ... Dr. Bruenn was an extremely thorough

12 In a 2008 telephone conversation with the author, Craig's nephew referred to the neurosurgeon as "Uncle Wink" and was unaware of any connection between him and FDR.

13 The president's T-shirt disappeared after the operation, and even though the entire operating room staff was restricted to base for a considerable length of time, Webster complained that it was never found. The mystery was solved by a most improbable twist of fate. While at a pulp magazine convention in Dayton, Ohio, in 2008, the author was casually conversing in the hotel bar with another of the attendees, John Gunnison, who told me he had grown up in Bethesda, Maryland. By virtue of my interest in Roosevelt's health I began telling him the story of the bloody T-shirt and to my profound shock, he replied, "I have the shirt in my house." I had serendipitously been speaking to the only person on earth who could have provided the solution! As it turned out, Gunnison's father, R. (Rolla) Harry Gunnison, was a pharmacist's mate assigned to Bethesda and one of his jobs was to put together the packets of drugs that FDR used while traveling. He had been in the operating room and purloined the T-shirt, eventually smuggling it out of his locker. Mrs. Gunnison was not thrilled at the prospect of housing a bloody shirt and laundered it. John happily supplied me with photos of his father's favorite souvenir. Harry Gunnison died in the 1970s. The details of the lists of medication he packed for FDR and the stories they might have told have been lost to history.

14 Shortly after the publication of *FDR's Deadly Secret* in 2010, I received a call from a physician In Michigan who told me his ex-wife, a pediatrician practicing in Rhode Island, was in possession of an original pathological slide from the February 1944 operation at Bethesda. When I contacted her, she told me her father had been a pathologist there and kept the slide (his prized possession), which she had inherited. She didn't know exactly where the slide was but would call me back when she found it. A few minutes later the phone rang after she had located it. It was labeled, "Franklin Delano Roosevelt, February 2, 1944, epidermoid cyst."

internist and cardiologist of high repute. I am sure he knows as much as it is possible to know about the President's health."

Daisy, who was in the dark at the time about any heart problems, declared "everything went off beautifully," adding that "the P., by all accounts, instructed the doctors as they worked."[15] Both she and Franklin were surprised that the eight stitches required to close the incision were covered only by a light gauze dressing. "[Franklin] had already concocted a story for the press about being like the Spirit of '76, with a big bandage around his head," Webster wrote.[16]

Two days later, Franklin brought up the operation at his regular news conference. Again, he joked. "Steve [Early] came in yesterday with blood in his eye," Franklin quipped to general laughter, describing how his press secretary had repeatedly been awakened after midnight to be asked "if [I] had been under the knife. That was the headline desired. And I said, 'Sure, I was under the knife. I am under the knife whenever I cut my fingernails.'" Franklin called the procedure "a preventative." "I don't know why I should talk about this," he said. "Mr. President, did those Naval 'gims' permit you to smoke while they did their hacking?" a reporter asked. "No," Franklin replied, "but I yelled for a cigarette right afterward." His audience laughed and moved on to a political subject.

The newspapers, if they mentioned the operation at all, ran short articles like one in *The New York Times* under a one-column headline, "Went Under Surgery, Roosevelt Discloses/But It Was Only For an Old Wen On His Head, He Says."[17] The account in the *Washington Post* was but two paragraphs, headlined "Roosevelt Recovers From Minor Surgery."[18] No one in the press raised any further questions about the operation.

Over the following weeks, Daisy Suckley noted Franklin was experiencing headaches and never-ending exhaustion. By the third week in March, she was fretting that "he finds it very hard to relax, unless he just falls asleep, sometimes sitting bolt upright,"[19] a good indication Franklin's heart failure had worsened—despite digitalis. During this period, Franklin often took to bed during the day and canceled appointments. "Every morning, in response to

---

15 *Suckley Diary*, February 2, 1944.
16 Webster to Goldsmith, Goldsmith, 52.
17 *New York Times*, February 5, 1944.
18 *Washington Post*, February 5, 1944.
19 *Suckley Diary*, March 23, 1944.

inquiry as to how he felt, a characteristic reply has been 'rotten,' or 'like hell,'" his personal secretary William Hassett wrote.[20] Grace Tully grew concerned about something she had never seen before. "I found the Boss occasionally nodding over his work or dozing a moment during dictation," she wrote. "He would grin in slight embarrassment as he caught himself ... but as it began to occur with increasing frequency I became seriously alarmed."[21] These events were epileptic seizures, though Tully, as many others who wrote and spoke about witnessing similar events, did not comprehend the medical significance to what she was seeing.

On March 20, 1944, Franklin was forced to cancel a meeting with Churchill in Bermuda, delaying a discussion of the final details of the invasion of France.

"R-506: FDR to WSC[22]

Washington (via U.S. Navy)

March 20, 1944, 6:30 p.m.

Personal and Secret. From the President for the Former Naval Person"

The strikethroughs are Franklin's, a rare window into his thinking.

"Replying to your 624 and in reference to your suggestion that we have a staff meeting on the Tehran scale in Bermuda about the fifth of April, it is not now possible for me to meet that date.

"Not having had any opportunity for relaxation since my recent attack of grippe which has not been completely eliminated leaves me from time to time with a temperature.

"My doctor considers it I ~~am very angry with myself. The old attack of grippe having hung on and on, leaving me with an intermittent temperature, Ross decided about a week ago that it is~~ necessary for me to take a complete rest of about two to three weeks in a suitable climate which I am definitely planning to do at the end of the month. I see no way out and I am furious."

Taking himself to task was another of Franklin's tells when he was hiding the truth.

---

20 Hassett, W., *Off the Record with FDR*, 239 (Diary entry for March 24, 1944.).

21 Tully, 274.

22 Kimball, W., ed., *Churchill and Roosevelt: The Complete Correspondence*, v. 3, Princeton, NJ: Princeton University Press, 1987, 59–60.

"It will therefore be impossible for me to get to a staff meeting in early April. I believe that such a meeting on the Tehran scale in early April would be most useful and if you agree I will send my Chiefs of Staff to Bermuda for that purpose at any time that suits your conveniences.

"I am glad that you feel hardened about Overlord. Its accomplishment may synchronize with a real Russian break-through."

The prime minister's response reveals Franklin had also planned to be in England on D-Day.

"C-629

WSC to FDR

London (via U.S. Army)

March 21, 1944, 1516 Z/TOR 1655 Z

Prime Minister to President Roosevelt. Most Secret and Personal.

Your 506

1   I am indeed grieved and trust rest will do you good.

2   I do not think the staff meeting worthwhile without our being there.

3   I hope you are still planning your visit here for the great event after you are fully recovered."

Franklin was also preparing for another important event at Hyde Park, a visit from Lucy Mercer on March 26 to show her around the library and Top Cottage.[23] He spent the previous day getting as much rest as possible in preparation for the visit, admitting to Daisy Suckley he was furious with himself. "I've never done such a thing in my life before," he told her, "Robert Louis Stevenson in the last days of consumption [tuberculosis]."

By March, Howard Bruenn was likely confronted with a big problem. Franklin's heart failure and arrhythmia were worsening and digitalis was not keeping them under control. Lacking other pharmacologic options, a decision was made to get him away from Washington to a place where rest could be enforced. On April 9, Franklin was taken to Hobcaw Barony, the coastal Georgetown, South Carolina estate of Wall Street magnate Bernard Baruch.[24]

---

23 Ward, *Closest Companion*, 287.
24 It is probably not coincidental that Franklin's close friend Cary Grayson had also stayed at

```
SA Reilly          The White House    Mar. 23,1944.
Chief              Washington,D.C.        President's trip.

    For your confidential information, you are advised that I conferred
with the President on this date and he has approved the following
schedule:

        Leave Washington. . . . . . . . . . 10:30 p.m., March 30.

        Arrive Morrison Field,
            West Palm Beach, Florida. . . . 1:30 a.m., April 1.

        Depart Morrison Field,
            West Palm Beach, Florida. . . .10:00 a.m., April 1.

        Arrive Guantanamo Base . . . . . . . . 1:05 p.m., April.

    His plans for the return to Washington and his means of travel
are still indefinite.  He has directed me to inquire into the
possibility of flying directly from Guantanamo Base to the most suitable
field nearest Warm Springs, Georgia, where if he returns by Warm Springs,
he would entrain for Washington, D. C.

                                    M. F. Reilly,
                                    Supervising Agent.
```

*Original Secret Service itinerary dated March 23, 1944 showing
original destination of Guantanamo Bay, Cuba.*

He had been told he needed "complete rest" about March 13 and had written to Churchill about it on March 20. The original destination had been Guantanamo Bay, Cuba, as confirmed by the Secret Service itinerary drawn up on March 23.[25]

The document also reveals Franklin's intention to follow his stay in Cuba with a visit to Warm Springs. The most likely explanation for the change in venue was a veto of air travel by cardiologist Bruenn—it was far too risky for his critically ill patient to fly. Another factor may have been the proximity of Hobcaw to Lucy Rutherfurd's home, 175 miles away in Aiken.

Hobcaw in 1936 to gain strength for an operation at the Mayo Clinic for lymphoma. Cary Grayson Papers, Staunton, VA.

25 Trips of the President.

At Hobcaw, Franklin abrogated nearly all his presidential duties to his chief of staff, Admiral William Leahy, and spent most of his time sleeping, fishing, and socializing with Lucy, who was lodged nearby.[26]

"The routine at Hobcaw showed how weak Roosevelt had become and how much he had grown to rely on Leahy," historian Phillips Payson O'Brien wrote in 2019. "After an early breakfast, Leahy would review all the top-secret dispatches sent to the president. He would answer some on his own, disregard others, and decide which few were so important that they needed to be discussed personally with Roosevelt. The president rose late—his plan during the trip was to sleep 12 hours a day—and was unable to start work until noon—at which point he and Leahy went through the messages Leahy had selected. For about an hour they would make decisions and plan responses before Roosevelt's workday was done and lunch was served.

"The early afternoon saw the president resting for a few more hours, until approximately 4 o'clock, when the party usually went for an excursion.... Leahy usually sat next to Roosevelt, at the president's insistence. Once back, they would enjoy an early dinner, followed by a movie or a game of cards. Roosevelt typically retired to bed not long after dinner was over."[27]

All of this remained secret until 2019. Leahy had written in his 1950 memoir, *I Was There*, that after Hobcaw, FDR "had regained his normal condition of health and was displaying some of his accustomed energy."[28]

Hypertension began playing a larger role in Franklin's medical history at this time and the subject needed to be put into historical perspective. The term "essential hypertension" was coined in 1911 to describe elevated blood pressure for which no cause could be found.[29] The potential for it to produce medical problems was not discussed until 1928, when a group of Mayo Clinic physicians described "malignant hypertension" as "a syndrome of very high blood pressure, damage to the retina of the eye and inadequate kidney function which often resulted in death within a year from strokes, heart fail-

26 Winik, J., *1944: FDR and The Year That Changed History.* New York: Simon & Schuster, 2016, 127.
27 O'Brien, P.P. *The Second Most Powerful Man in the World.* New York: Dutton, 2019. 270–271.
28 Leahy, W., *I Was There.* New York: Whittlesey House, 1950, 237.
29 For an excellent review of the history of hypertension see: Kotchen, T.A., "Historical Trends and Milestones in Hypertension Research a Model of the Process of Translational Research." *Hypertension*, 2011;58:522–538.

ure or kidney failure." This sounds very much like the "Bright's Disease" that killed Ellen Axson Wilson in 1914. The Mayo team's definition of "very high" was a diastolic pressure (the lower number) exceeding 120.[30]

In 1931, John Hay, professor of medicine at Liverpool University, wrote: "There is some truth in the saying that the greatest danger to a man with a high blood pressure lies in its discovery, because then some fool is certain to try and reduce it."[31] This view was shared by America's preeminent cardiologist, Paul Dudley White, who wrote in 1937, "Hypertension may be an important compensatory mechanism which should not be tampered with, even if we were certain that we could control it."[32] Until 1949, the consensus of the medical community was that blood pressure under 210/100 was not dangerous.[33]

In modern terms, Franklin's blood pressure in April 1944 was severely elevated—as documented in a log kept by George Fox at Hobcaw. There were many days, particularly in the last half of the month, when the president would have been rushed off to a present-day emergency room.[34]

Even if Bruenn had wanted to treat Franklin's hypertension, his options were limited to a bland diet, toxic cyanide compounds, and sedatives. The first effective drug to lower blood pressure was not introduced until 1950.[35] Diuretics (water pills), now a standard treatment, did not appear until 1958.

On April 25, Eleanor and Anna flew to Hobcaw from Washington with John Curtin, the Prime Minister of Australia, for lunch and returned to Washington later in the day.[36]

"Late in the afternoon [of April 28] [Franklin] began to complain of abdominal pain and tenderness associated with slight nausea," Bruenn wrote in 1970, "There were no cardiac symptoms ... A tentative diagnosis of acute

---

30 Keith, N.M., Wagener, H.P., Kernohan, N.M., "The Syndrome of Malignant Hypertension." *Archives Intern Medicine* 1928;41(2):141–188.

31 Hay, J., "A British Medical Journal Association Lecture on the Significance of a Raised Blood Pressure." *British Medical Journal* July 1931;2(3679):43–47.

32 White, P.D., *Heart Disease* (2nd ed.). New York: MacMillan Co., 1937, 326.

33 Friedberg, C.K. *Diseases of the Heart*. Philadelphia, PA: WB Saunders Co., 1949.

34 *Howard Bruenn Papers*, FDRL. Some of the recordings were taken on the days that Bruenn was in Washington.

35 Hydralazine, a vasodilator, was discovered in 1949. Reserpine, a depleter of epinephrine-like substances, came into use in 1955.

36 FDR Day by Day, April 24, 1944.

```
                          WASHINGTON, D.C.
                          April 9, 1944

9th    202/102   P.M.   196/96

10th   196/94     "     200/104

11th   192/96     "     204/100

12th   200/102    "     204/98

13th   198/100    "     202/98

14th   206/100    "     200/96

15th   206/102    "     196/100

16th   215/102    "     206/120

17th   216/120    "     206/116 (Dr.Bruen 4th sound)

18th   220/120 (4th sound) Unicap 1; KI x x t.i.d. sc.

19th   218/120   P.M.   204/104

20th   212/108   Noon 210/98   9:54 p.m. 190/100 (KI discontinued)

21st   9:05 a.m. 234/126; 10:a.m. (sitting) 210/116; 10:05 a.m. 2
       (prone, both arms checked) 6:45 p.m. after outing 214/120;
       9:50 p.m. 220/114.

22nd   9:30 a.m. 214/ 120;  11:30 a.m. 210/114; 6:30 p.m.
       (after boat trip) 208/110.

23rd   10:15 a.m. 214/118 (2½ hr drive)  9:45 212/114.

24th   10:a.m. 222/122  10:30 p.m. 220/116

25th   10:05  224/116  10 p.m. 214/106 (after luncheon party).

26th   10. a.m. 214/112  10;30 p.m. 222/110

27th   10:15 a.m. 222/118;  9:45 p.m. 210/114

28th   224/124     P.M. 230/120  (one additional digit tablet
                                  Tuesday and Friday)

29th   9:a.m. (on awaking) 196/112;(sitting after breakfast) 10;1
       236/120;  (Prone, after E.K.) 220/118;  2:15 (after lunch)
       236/112 (Thesodate discontinued)  9:30 p.m. 210/110

30th   8:45 (Prone, on awaking) 210/110;(after breakfast) 10:00
       206/104;  ; after lunch 208/114;  9:00 p.m. 234/120

May 1st. Prone 9:a.m. 220/116; Noon 210/110; 2 p.m. (after lunch
       210/ 106;  10:30 p.m. 210/112.
```

Log of FDRs blood pressures while at Hobcaw Barony, April 1944.

165

cholecystitis [gallstones] was made, and he was given codeine by hypodermic injection, with some relief. He slept well, but the next day the symptoms were still present ... [H]e was put on a soft diet. By May 1 he was free of all abdominal distress ... and appeared to be in good shape. Because of his apparent recovery, normal diet was resumed, but after luncheon on May 2 he had a recurrence of his abdominal distress and that evening was acutely uncomfortable."[37]

Abdominal pain of this nature was the bailiwick of Dr. Lahey, a world-class surgeon who was well-versed in the case. Lahey Clinic surgeon David Preston Boyd later wrote in an unpublished history of that facility, which has mysteriously disappeared, that it was "beyond the outposts of reason for Lahey not to almost certainly have been consulted when Roosevelt suffered an acute abdomen [medical-speak for an unexplained attack of severe stomach pain] ... The strange disappearance of [Franklin's medical records] is only one of the enigmas of the President's last illness.[38] It says to all in thunderous tones: 'Much was hidden,'" Boyd wrote. "To contemplate Frank H. Lahey as a partner in a cover-up is almost beyond the capability of those who knew him best and are still here to justify; but all can see the circumstances were unique. That Lahey would certify as fit and well a man who he considered a threat to the country's economic life and to the safety of the world *and in whom he found a terminal malignancy* (emphasis added) is to pull the snout of reason. But he may have done it."[39]

Harry Goldsmith, himself a highly respected surgeon, wrote in 2005, "It seems difficult to believe that the acute abdominal pain suffered by FDR for a week was not addressed by at least one consulting surgeon as warranted by the potentially catastrophic progression that this serious abdominal condition can pose ... Dr. Lahey had examined FDR in Washington shortly before his gall bladder attack, and it seems logical if a surgical consultant was needed in South Carolina it would almost certainly would have been Dr. Lahey."[40]

Daisy Suckley arrived at Hobcaw on May 4. "Under his tan, FDR looks thin & drawn & not a bit well," she wrote. "He is on a strict diet, feels good-for-nothing, has just had some sort of an 'attack' which seems to be in the upper part of the

---

37 Bruenn, 584.
38 As is the strange disappearance of Boyd's manuscript!
39 Goldsmith, 37.
40 *Ibid.*, Goldsmith reviewed a 22-page chapter from Boyd's unpublished history of the Lahey Clinic. The manuscript has disappeared.

abdomen. He says they don't know what is the matter with him—I wonder if perhaps they don't want to tell him." The abdominal pain was Franklin's second attack in South Carolina. The episode occurred the day after Bruenn had returned to Hobcaw from Bethesda, after spending two days collaborating with Dr. Paul Dudley White in Washington to treat Navy Secretary Frank Knox's ultimately fatal heart attack. No doubt Franklin's heart disease had been a topic of discussion between the two eminent cardiologists.[41] Franklin was too ill to attend Knox's funeral and sent "Pa" Watson in his place.

An incomplete letter to Daisy, handwritten in pencil by Franklin, reveals his awareness of his cardiac problem.[42] "I am really feeling 'no good'—don't want to do anything & want to sleep all the time," he wrote. "I forgot to tell you that Dr. Bruin [sic] came down, too—He is one of the best heart men—Tho' my own is definitely better—does queer things still."[43] On May 5, Daisy confirmed what the "queer things" were—atrial fibrillation, a significant and potentially life-threatening cardiac arrhythmia.

"Downstairs at 10, [Franklin] had had a good night & looked better … Dr. Bruenn came along & I talked about the P. He relieved me by saying the P's blood is all right, I had feared the trouble he had two years ago.[44] From a later talk with the P. the trouble is evidently with his heart—*the diastole & systole are not working properly in unison*—but there is definite improvement.

"I had a good talk with the P. about himself. He said he had discovered that the doctors had not agreed together about what to tell him, so that he found out that they were not telling him the whole truth & that he was evidently more sick than they said! It is foolish of them to attempt to put anything over on *him!*"[45]

---

41 Secretary of the Navy Frank Knox was admitted to the Naval Hospital at Bethesda with a severe heart attack. With Bruenn tending to Franklin in South Carolina, White was called in. As the hospital's chief of cardiology, Bruenn was obliged to join White in Bethesda to co-treat the naval secretary. Nursing notes confirm the two doctors were together. They were unable to save Knox's life. Knox medical records, Ross McIntire files, FDRL.
42 The letter wound up in the cache of papers Daisy left to be found in 1991 and now resides in the collection of Roosevelt House in New York City. Geoffrey Ward described it as being written in "an alarmingly shaky hand." Actually, the letter no different than Franklin's other writing while using a pencil. Ward, *Closest Companion*, 295.
43 *Ibid.*
44 This appears to be a reference to the anemia first diagnosed on May 5, 1941.
45 *Ibid.*, 298.

Franklin and Daisy returned to Washington on May 7. "I am really practically all right again though I am still having some tests made on my plumbing and am keeping regular hours with much allocation to sleep." Franklin wrote Churchill on May 20. "The old bronchial pneumonia [in truth, congestive heart failure] has completely disappeared. The real triumph is that I have lost nearly ten pounds in the last couple of months and now I have begun the struggle to maintain the loss.[46]

"I do not believe I can get away for over a month. Of course, I am greatly disappointed that I could not be in England just at this moment [referring to D-day,] or perhaps having missed the boat it will be best not to make the trip until the events of the near future are more clear."[47]

Though Franklin had spent a month sequestered from the press and public, his health problems continued to escape most Americans. "According to the reporters who have seen him, the President comes back to Washington bronzed, rested and fit," columnist Anne O'Hare McCormick wrote in *The New York Times*. "Only a man of extraordinary temperament and resilience could have weathered as buoyantly as he has done during the continual and ever-accelerating crisis he has presided over."[48]

Harold Ickes was now worried that the president had too few appointments to transact any meaningful business. "It seems that [Franklin] had some trouble with his colon, which at first he thought might be a growth [cancer, in layman's parlance]," Ickes wrote on May 20. "Then it suddenly moved to his left side under his heart. It was very painful. Then, without notice, it moved clear over to his right side, where it again caused him pain. At any rate, this had the effect of persuading him that it could not be a growth. Then suddenly it disappeared and he had no pain. He is going to the Naval Hospital soon to have a complete checkup."[49]

---

46 This is the only record of Franklin personally stating he wanted to maintain a low weight. His weight problem would soon be of the opposite nature.
47 Kimball, W., ed. *Churchill & Roosevelt. The Complete Correspondence. III. Alliance Declining. February 1944 – April 1945.* Princeton, NJ: Princeton University Press, 1984;R-542/1:139.
48 *New York Times*, May 8, 1944.
49 *Ickes' Diary*, May 20, 1944.

The May 25 Suckley diary entry describes the unmistakable preparatory regimen for a test to visualize the gall bladder. The test on May 26 allegedly revealed "a small group of cholesterol stones"[50] but no report has surfaced.

The Normandy invasion, scheduled for June 4, was postponed due to unfavorable weather. On June 5, Rome fell to the Allies. At 3 a.m. on June 6, the White House switchboard called Eleanor to wake her husband. Franklin got no more sleep that night as bulletins from General George Marshall at the War Department poured in from France. Early reports indicated lighter than expected casualties. By day's end, Allied troops had established a critical beachhead. Franklin's radio address to the nation that evening included a prayer.

---

50 Bruenn, H.G., "Clinical Notes on the Illness and Death of President Franklin D. Roosevelt." *Annals of Internal Medicine*, 1970;72(4):579–591, 580.

■ Chapter 21
■ The Last Campaign

Franklin's pursuit of a fourth term was universally acknowledged as a given, especially after the success of the D-Day invasion and that summer's hard-fought breakout across Nazi-occupied Europe. Secretary of Labor, Frances Perkins, wrote that no one in the cabinet feared health concerns would keep him from running.[1] But Harold Ickes and the new Navy Secretary, James Forrestal, both felt Franklin would probably not serve out a fourth term. "I don't necessarily mean that the president will die in office or become so incapacitated that he might not be capable of carrying on," Ickes wrote. "He might very well resign. I believe that he is sick of domestic affairs and after the war would like to devote himself exclusively to the world situation."[2]

There were no serious challengers for the nomination, but a chorus of skepticism about his fitness to serve resounded. After dining with Franklin at the White House in late March 1944, founding director of the National Youth Administration Aubrey Williams told *The New York Times* the president "looked so tired and worn that I was shocked." Williams said he had "the distinct impression that [Franklin] wouldn't run again, although he didn't say so directly."[3]

As he had been in 1940, Franklin was coy about his plans. "I haven't even decided if I will run," he told Daisy in May. "What will decide for me ... will be the way I feel in a couple of months. If I know I am not going to be able to carry on for another four years, it wouldn't be fair to the American people to run for another term," he said.[4] On June 20, Daisy, who never questioned anything Franklin told her, wrote, "the P. doesn't know if he will run or not."[5]

Eleanor knew better. "I knew without asking that as long as the war was on, it was a foregone conclusion that Franklin, if he was well enough, would run

---

1 Perkins, 388.
2 *Ickes Diary*, June 4, 1944.
3 *New York Times*, March 26, 1944.
4 *Suckley Diary*, May 22, 1944.
5 *Ibid.*, June 20, 1944.

again," she recalled.[6] "The people elected me their leader and I can't quit in the middle of the war," Franklin told his son John.[7]

Fatalism began creeping into Franklin's interactions. "Here is something you ought to write if I should pop off," he told press aide Jonathan Daniels, the son of Josephus, Franklin's mentor during the Wilson administration.[8] United Press White House correspondent Merriman Smith began to notice an uncharacteristic lack of vigor. At news conferences "he became listless and poor of voice," Smith wrote. "He reached the point where he lost enthusiasm for denouncing certain irritant correspondents as liars."[9] Even his trusted personal aide, General "Pa" Watson, complained that the president "just doesn't seem to give a damn."[10]

At Hyde Park Franklin "slept late, retired early, and took no afternoon drives," biographer Jim Bishop wrote. "The deep, mottled gray under Roosevelt's eyes seemed to be blackish in certain light; the President tired of wheeling himself from ground floor office to upstairs room, and the work of pushing the chair was undertaken by a Secret Service man who noted the scrawny neck and the nodding head ... the hands, except when at rest on the edge of a desk, trembled more than previously."[11]

New Deal "top brain" Benjamin V. Cohen told Franklin that a fourth term would be "anticlimactic." Cohen suggested a deal to get the Democratic and Republican presidential nominees to agree to establish the United Nations with him as chief executive officer.[12]

"That is a tremendously interesting analysis—and I think a very just one," Franklin responded. "You have only left out one matter—and that is the matter of my own feelings!"[13]

---

6 Bishop, J. *FDR's Last Year April 1944–April 1945*. New York: William Morrow & Company, 1974, 72.

7 Gallagher, 193.

8 Daniels, J., *White House Witness 1942–1945*. New York: Doubleday, 1975, 220.

9 Smith, M., *Thank You, Mr. President*. New York: Harper & Brothers, 1946, 25.

10 Lash, J.P., Eleanor and Franklin: The Story of Their Relationship, Based on Eleanor Roosevelt's Private Papers. New York: W.W Norton, 1971, 709.

11 Bishop, 83.

12 *Ibid.*, 22–23.

13 *Ibid.*

On July 28, *Life* asked Ross McIntire whether Franklin could survive a fourth term. "The President's health is excellent. I can say that unqualifiedly,"[14] McIntire answered. "With proper care and strict adherence to rules, I gave it as my best judgment that his chances of winning through to 1948 were *good.* [emphasis in original]," But McIntire covered himself by saying he had told the president "unless he slowed down, I would not be answerable for the consequences."[15] All this despite his patient being just sixty-two years old and supposedly in the best of health.

The presidential physician had secretly conveyed the opposite message three weeks earlier. On July 8, McIntire, Frank Lahey, and James Paullin evaluated FDR and Lahey memorialized their assessment in a private document. "The Lahey Memorandum," remained a closely guarded secret for more than four decades.

> "I wish to record the following information regarding my opinions in relation to President Roosevelt's condition and to have them on record in the event there comes any criticism of me at a later date," Lahey wrote. "I want to do this after having seen him in consultation as a private record.
>
> "On Saturday July 8, I talked with Admiral McIntire in my capacity as one of the group of three, Admiral McIntire, Dr. James Paullin of Atlanta, Georgia, and myself who saw President Roosevelt in consultation and who have been over his physical examination, x-rays, and laboratory findings concerning his physical condition. I have reviewed all of his x-rays over the past years and compared them with all the present findings and am recording my opinion concerning Mr. Roosevelt's condition and capacities now. I am recording these opinions in the light of having informed Admiral McIntire Saturday afternoon July 8, 1944 that I did not believe that, if Mr. Roosevelt was elected President again, he had the physical capacity to complete a term. I told him that, as a result of activities in his trip to Russia[16] he had been in a state which was, if not in heart failure, at least on the verge of it, that this was the result of high blood pressure he has had now for a long time, plus a question of coronary damage. With this in mind it was my opinion that over the four years of another term with its burdens, he would again have heart failure and be unable to complete it. Admiral McIntire was in agreement with this.

---

14 "The President's Doctor." *Life*, July 28, 1944.
15 McIntire, 193.
16 The only trip Roosevelt ever made to "Russia,"(actually the U.S.S.R.) was the summit meeting at Yalta, which took place six months after this memo was written. Lahey probably meant the Tehran conference, which took place the previous November.

"In addition to that I stated that it was not my duty to advise concerning whether or not such a term was undertaken, but to inform Admiral McIntire, as his family Physician, that it was my opinion that it was Admiral McIntire's duty to inform him concerning his capacity.

"In addition to the above I have told Admiral McIntire that I feel strongly that if he does accept another term, he has a very serious responsibility concerning who is the Vice President. Admiral McIntire agreed with this and has, he states, so informed Mr. Roosevelt.

"I am putting this on record. I am asking that it be witnessed, sealed and placed in safekeeping. It is to be opened and utilized only in the event that there might be criticism of me should this later eventuate and the criticisms be directed toward me for not having made this public. As I see my duty as a physician, I cannot violate my professional position nor possible professional confidence, but I do wish to be on record concerning possible later criticism.

Frank M. Lahey"

Witness

L.M. Strand[17]

The witness to the exculpatory memorandum was Linda Strand, who was as close to Lahey as Missy LeHand had been to Franklin. Upon his death in 1953, Lahey left control of half the value of his clinic to Strand. She and Dr. Harry S. Goldsmith successfully sued to gain the release of the memo in 1985 but its contents were not made public by Goldsmith until 2005 in his self-published book, *Conspiracy of Silence*. Despite an abundance of subsequent Roosevelt biographies, neither the historical implications of the Lahey memorandum nor many other important details of Franklin's illnesses that Goldsmith unearthed, have been incorporated into the narrative of Franklin's health— with the notable exception of *FDR's Deadly Secret* in 2010.[18]

The memorandum was drafted primarily out of Lahey's concern for his reputation, but confirms that doctors concurred that Franklin would not survive a fourth term. Bruenn was surely in the mix. A surgeon of Lahey's stature would never have offered a prognosis outside his specialty without the input and consent of the president's cardiologist.

17 Goldsmith, 171–172.
18 Lomazow, S., Fettmann, E. *FDR's Deadly Secret*. New York: Public Affairs, 2010.

The memo is silent on the subject of cancer. Skeptics point to this as an indication that Franklin did not have a malignancy—but this assumption flies in the face of repeated credible firsthand reports from reputable physicians, several of them close associates of Lahey, who quote him as reporting that the president had cancer.[19] Cancers were Franklin's deepest secrets. The document was fashioned such that if it were made public at a later date, the cancer cover-up would not be exposed.[20] Howard Bruenn clearly had this is mind when he wrote his 1970 medical paper.

Franklin's horrendous prognosis did not alter McIntire's public stance. An article in *Life* on July 31, 1944, implied he had told the president the exact opposite. "[W]hen President Roosevelt announced that he would run for a fourth term, it was not a wholly personal decision," the magazine wrote. "The person who presumably made up the president's mind was not Harry Hopkins, [Democratic national committee chairman] Robert Hannegan, or even Mrs. Roosevelt, but Vice Admiral Ross T. McIntire, surgeon general of the United States Navy, official White House physician and vigilant watchdog over the chief executive's health."[21] McIntire stated that a determining factor in Roosevelt's decision to seek a fourth term was his physical condition, and that he did not announce his candidacy until he was assured that his health was adequate to the task.

Franklin was also undeterred. The day after being told he would not survive a fourth term, he wrote Hannegan, "reluctantly, but as a good soldier ... I will accept and serve in the office, if I am so ordered by the Commander-in-Chief of us all—the sovereign people of the United States."[22]

The Democratic National Convention convened on July 19, 1944. There was widespread whispered consensus that Franklin's running mate was destined to become president. Eleanor supported Vice President Henry Wallace, but party leaders vigorously opposed him as, among other glaring liabilities, being too liberal. "I could make no greater individual contribution to the nation's

---

19 Lahey has been quoted by multiple physicians including Dr. George Pack that Franklin had "stomach cancer." Some have been more specific, stating that he had liver metastases.
20 In his response to readers of the journal that published "Clinical Notes," Bruenn had gone so far as to lie that McIntire had probably never told Roosevelt how severely ill he was. Lerner, BH. "Crafting Medical History: Revisiting the 'Definitive' Account of Franklin D. Roosevelt's Terminal Illness." *Bulletin of the History of Medicine* Summer 2007;81(2):386–406, footnote 48.
21 Perkins, J. "The President's Doctor." *Life* July 31, 1944;17:4, quoted in Goldsmith, 43.
22 Lomazow and Fettmann, 123.

good than to do everything in my power to protect it from Wallace during the war and postwar period," Democratic Party Treasurer Edwin Pauley declared. "My pre-convention slogan was, 'You are not nominating a Vice-President of the United States, but a President.'"[23]

Franklin wasn't about to distract from his goal of establishing the United Nations by endorsing a controversial running mate. "I am just not going to go through a convention like 1940 again," he told Sam Rosenman. "It will split the party wide open, and it is already split enough between North and South; it may kill our chances for election this fall, and if it does, it will prolong the war and knock into a cocked hat all the plans we've been making for the future."[24]

Rosenman and Ickes sat Wallace down and told him in no uncertain terms he had become a political liability, but the vice president insisted he was still going to fight for the job. Wallace went directly to Franklin, arguing that he was the only one who could keep the Black vote in the Democratic column, given his outspokenness on civil rights and Black leaders' disappointment at Franklin's refusal to integrate the armed forces. Wallace announced that Franklin told him, "I hope it's the same team again, Henry,"[25] but this was nothing more than Franklin's characteristic ploy of never giving anyone bad news to their face. He used the same maneuver with Dixiecrat Jimmy Byrnes of South Carolina, encouraging him to run though well aware of the disqualifying distaste union, Black, and Catholic voters had for Byrnes.[26] Privately, Franklin's first choice for vice president was Supreme Court Justice William O. Douglas.[27] He had also flirted with the idea of tapping steel magnate Henry Kaiser.[28]

Another recurring name was Senator Harry Truman, Robert Hannegan's fellow Missourian. Truman had distinguished himself as chairman of a commission

23 Pauley memorandum, Harry S. Truman Library.

24 Rosenman, S., *Working with Roosevelt*. London: Rupert Hart-Davis, 1952, 439.

25 Bishop, 100.

26 Byrnes was an avowed racist and had actively opposed anti-lynching legislation. He had also abandoned his Catholic faith to marry. The story was one of Franklin's favorite cocktail hour anecdotes.

27 Columnist Jack Anderson also revealed in 1987 that "shortly before he died, Justice William O. Douglas told him that FDR had given Democratic National Chairman Robert Hannegan two choices to replace Vice President Henry Wallace in the 1944 election. Douglas was FDR's first choice, Sen. Harry S Truman his second. But he knew Truman was more acceptable to the politicians, so he reversed the order of names when he passed them on to the convention, which dutifully nominated Truman." "Evidence FDR Knew of Cancer" Anderson, J., Spear, J., *Washington Post*, July 2, 1987.

28 *Suckley Diary*, May 22, 1944.

to reduce waste and inefficiency in military spending. He denied any interest at first. Throughout American history, so-called "'accidental presidents' were ridiculed in office, had their hearts broken, lost any vestige of respect they had before. I don't want that to happen to me," Truman told his daughter Margaret.[29] He even agreed to nominate Byrnes for the slot. It looked like Byrnes might be the nominee until powerful labor leaders Sidney Hillman and Phillip Murray told the Dixiecrat point blank they could not back him under any circumstances.

Truman was the candidate least likely to arouse serious opposition, so Franklin phoned Hannegan at the convention in Chicago. With Truman reportedly listening in, the president asked, "Have you got that fellow lined up yet?"

"Not yet," Hannegan replied.

"Tell the senator that if he wants to break up the Democratic Party by staying out, he can," Franklin said. "But he knows as well as I what that might mean at this dangerous time in the world."[30] Franklin followed up the call with a note indicating he'd be happy to run with either Douglas or Truman.

Because Franklin did not personally announce his choice, the delegates had heard mixed messages. Wallace led after the first ballot. On the second, some big states began switching to Truman and the stampede was on; Truman was nominated easily.

Franklin accepted the nomination over the radio on July 20, 1944, from his private railway car, *Ferdinand Magellan*, at a Marine Corps base near San Diego, Camp Pendleton. He and Eleanor had spent the previous six days on a cross-country, nonpolitical rail trip to visit their son James, who was stationed there as an intelligence officer.

Franklin was supposed to review Marine landing exercises on the morning of his acceptance speech—plans nearly waylaid when he was stricken with excruciating abdominal pain.[31] He mentioned the incident in a letter to Eleanor, who had left the previous day. "Jimmy and I had a grand view of

---

29 *Washington Post*, November 20, 1972.
30 *Ibid.*
31 The excruciating, short-duration abdominal pain manifested by Franklin is consistent with a telescoping of the small bowel due to a partial obstruction known as intussusception. It is a rare but well-recognized complication of metastatic melanoma.

the landing operation at Camp Pendleton and then I got the collywobbles & stayed in the train in the p.m.," he wrote. "Better today."[32]

Years later, James provided a chilling description of "the collywobbles." Father and son were alone in the private rail car, with doctors McIntire and Bruenn a shout away, when Franklin began to groan. "His face took on an expression of pain and suffering, and all the color seemed to drain from it," James wrote. "Jimmy, I don't know if I can make it. I have horrible pains, he exclaimed." James helped his father get down on the floor from his berth and offered to call the doctor. Franklin refused, insisting that the paralyzing abdominal pains were not from his heart but merely indigestion. "So for perhaps ten minutes, while I kept as quiet as possible, Father lay on the floor of his railroad car, his eyes closed, his face drawn, his powerful torso occasionally convulsed as the waves of pain stabbed him. Never in all my life had I felt so alone with him—and so helpless ... Then he opened his eyes, exhaled deeply, and said, 'Help me up now, Jimmy.' I did so. I helped him get ready, and the Commander-in-Chief went out to review the exercises."[33] Anna later attempted to discredit her brother's story by claiming he lacked the strength to lift his father out of his berth.

Many of the stories James told about his father are blatantly false, especially those set during the Easter 1934 cruise aboard *Nourmahal*. It is fair to be skeptical about anything he writes. But this event had been corroborated by Franklin and is reminiscent of episodes described by Charles Bohlen at Tehran and the two that occurred at Hobcaw. In this particular instance, James's account appears to be accurate.

Only hours after the attack, Franklin told the nation over the radio, "I shall not campaign, in the usual sense, for the office. In these days of tragic sorrow, I do not consider it fitting. And besides, in these days of global warfare, I shall not be able to find the time."[34] The speech revealed Democrats planned to depict the election as a choice between turning the presidency over "to inexperienced or immature hands"—GOP nominee Thomas E. Dewey was forty-two years old and had been governor of New York for less than two years—and leaving in charge "those who saw the danger from abroad, who met it head-on and who now have seized the offensive and carried the war to its present stages of

32 Bishop, 111.
33 Roosevelt and Shalett, 351–352.
34 *New York Times*, July 21, 1944.

success."[35] The strategy also blunted Dewey's ability to emphasize his youth and vigor in contrast to the president's visible physical deterioration.

A photo of Franklin delivering his acceptance speech in the July 31 issue of *Life* showed him glassy-eyed with his mouth agape. Harold Ickes said the image by staff photographer George Skadding made Franklin look "like a sitting ghost."[36,37] Robert G. Nixon, the White House correspondent of the International News Service, received an urgent call from his editor in New York. "My god, that photograph," said the editor. "Is Roosevelt dying?"[38]

Steve Early was furious. "I was terrifically disappointed, let down to a new low," he wrote to Grace Tully. "I can't imagine what was wrong with Skadding, or his camera, or his subject. But something decidedly was wrong ... The rumor factory is working overtime—making all it can out of rumors and lies about the President's health. That is why some of the photographs I have seen caused me so much concern."[39] *The New York Times* reported on July 22, "A photograph taken of him delivering this speech seemed to show a very haggard, ill, old man."[40]

Called on the carpet, Skadding explained he'd hurriedly turned his negatives over to the wire photo agencies. "They grabbed the first shot they looked at and before I knew it they had this particular bad shot on the wires."[41] As for the "terrible picture of the Boss" that his magazine published in its July 31 issue—with the strange gape and Franklin's extra-wide pants legs visible—"I felt like apologizing, but the dam [sic] picture's been used," he wrote. "I have already gripped [sic] like hell to my office—That kind of a shot does not do me any good. To try and make up for this I'm going to personally supervise the ones made and show the boss as he really is."[42]

Franklin's facial expression was not the only problem the photo created. Also in the picture were Franklin's son James flanked by two of his sisters-in-law. Another man in uniform appears in the foreground caught in profile—Howard

35 *Ibid.*
36 *Harold Ickes Diary*, August 6, 1944.
37 Lensman Skadding had apparently caught Franklin in the midst of a seizure.
38 Robert G. Nixon oral history, Harry S. Truman Library.
39 Steve Early to Grace Tully, July 28, 1944. Early papers FDRL-HP, quoted in Ferrell, R.H., *The Dying President*, 79.
40 *New York Times*, July 22, 1944.
41 George Skadding to Steve Early, August 2, 1944, Early papers, FDRL-HP.
42 *Ibid.*

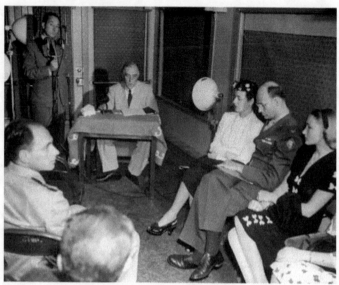

Life magazine photo probably showing FDR in the midst of a seizure. Howard Bruenn seen in profile in the left foreground.

Bruenn. Walter Trohan later wrote he had seen one of the wire service versions of the photo in which Bruenn's face had been cropped out, but noticed "the hand and lower sleeve of a naval commander. I couldn't imagine how so low-ranking an officer could be the only armed services guest at such a historic address." He requested a full-frame print of the original and took it to the Navy Department for identification. "I was told he was Commander Howard Bruenn," Trohan said. "Further inquiry revealed that he was a heart specialist."[43]

On August 6, 1944, The Chicago *Tribune* ran a story on page three under the headline "Disclose Heart Specialist Is With Roosevelt. President Roosevelt's health and stamina again became a major topic of capital conversation today with the disclosure that a heart specialist is a member of his official party." The story went on to identify the mystery officer. "It was reported in capital circles Bruenn has been commissioned to look after Mr. Roosevelt." The White House offered no comment. No other paper or wire service picked up the story.

43 Trohan, W., *Political Animals*, New York: Doubleday, 1975, 200.

But others did notice. There had long been scuttlebutt at Bethesda about Bruenn's frequent absences, which seemed to coincide with Franklin leaving town. The gossip intensified when someone at the hospital received a clipping of Trohan's story. Assistant Secretary of State Breckinridge Long got wind of the rumors and traced the mutterings to Colonel Byrl R. Kirklin, an Army Medical Corps radiology specialist who had worked at the Mayo Clinic before the war.

Long discovered that Kirklin had told a group of Mayo doctors the president had heart disease and "is going ahead anyhow and doing his regular job." Long reported his findings to Steve Early,[44] who gave the information to FBI director J. Edgar Hoover.[45] Within three days, the FBI had interviewed Kirklin and filed a report. They also interviewed Dr. Howard Odel at Bethesda Naval Medical Center, who had shown Kirklin a floor at the hospital reserved for high-ranking government officials. While the president had not stayed overnight, he "had been at the hospital on two or three occasions for examinations," Kirklin said. The FBI report revealed, "There had been rumors circulating about the President's health and [Kirklin] wondered if the president had heart disease or hypertension." He may have added something to the effect that "I suspect there may be something to it."[46] Hoover dismissed the story as gossip.[47]

On July 22, two days after accepting the nomination, Franklin boarded heavy cruiser USS *Baltimore* for Hawaii to meet with Admiral Chester Nimitz and General Douglas MacArthur to strategize the end-game of the Pacific war. Nimitz proposed a push westward, culminating in an invasion of the island of Formosa—the most direct path to the Japanese home islands. But the flamboyant MacArthur had vowed, "I shall return" upon being driven from the Philippines in 1942. The General demanded an attack on Luzon, the main Philippine island, where 7,000 American POWs were imprisoned, followed by an advance on Manila. "You cannot abandon seventeen million loyal Filipino Christians to the Japanese in favor of first liberating Formosa and returning it to China," MacArthur argued.[48] Franklin decided in favor of MacArthur after George Marshall, one of his most influential military advisers, endorsed his plan.

---

44 Breckinridge Long to Steve Early, October 29, 1944, Federal Bureau of Investigation.
45 Crispell and Gomez, 111.
46 "Memorandum Re: Circulation of Story Alleging the President has a Serious Heart Affliction," October 29, 1944, FBI.
47 J. Edgar Hoover to Stephen Early, November 1, 1944, FBI.
48 Lomazow and Fettmann, 131.

■ Chapter 22
■ A Rapidly Failing Candidate

Franklin left Hawaii aboard *Baltimore* on July 29, 1944, bound for the naval base at Adak, Alaska, arriving on August 3.[1] Four days later he boarded destroyer USS *Cummings* and docked at Puget Sound Navy Yard in Bremerton, Washington, on August 12. That afternoon he addressed 5,000 workers from the destroyer's forecastle deck. His remarks were broadcast nationwide. A film crew recorded the event.

Franklin intended the speech to be as a "homey report" of his trip, working only with Navy stenographer, William Rigdon. The Bremerton address turned out to be "one of the poorest speeches he made, both in form and in delivery," Grace Tully noted.[2] "People would be inclined to reason from this speech that the President was not a well man and that would not spell votes," Harold Ickes wrote.[3] "Others thought that the President's delivery indicated that he might have had an extra cocktail too much."[4,5] Assistant Secretary of War, John J. McCloy, a pro-FDR Republican, told Ickes that "his Republican friends might hesitate to vote for Roosevelt if his health was as the speech might seem to indicate." Listening on the radio, Sam Rosenman experienced "a sinking sensation." The president sounded "hesitant, halting, and indecisive. It was a dismal failure," he later wrote.[6] Daisy Suckley was also tuned in. "It seemed to me as though he was tired and that he once or twice got mixed up in his words. This would mean nothing with anyone else, but we expect perfection with the P. & any tiny slip of any kind always worries me!" she wrote on August 12. "I hope I am all wrong and that he is feeling wonderfully rested and benefited by the trip."[7]

---

1 This is the time when Republicans alleged Franklin had left Fala aboard the cruiser, which became the subject of his famous campaign speech to the Teamsters Union months later.
2 Tully, 198–199.
3 *Harold Ickes Diary*, August 12, 1944.
4 *Ibid.*
5 Knowing how FDR used alcohol as an anesthetic as he did at his fourth inauguration, the idea he might have had a few drinks prior to his speech is not far-fetched.
6 Rosenman, 62.
7 *Suckley Diary*, August 12, 1944.

An inspection tour around the Naval base was canceled.[8] Howard Bruenn later claimed Franklin had suffered an attack of angina pectoris—chest pain from coronary insufficiency—while speaking. Film reveals no overt discomfort and disproves later suggestions by Bruenn that the wind was playing havoc with Franklin's script and the destroyer's deck was pitching.[9]

A reasonable alternative explanation for the pain is spinal bone metastases, a frequent and dreaded consequence of prostate cancer. Franklin had not stood in his leg braces for over a year. Bruenn hinted at the problem on April 23, when his notes reveal that Franklin was using "an abdominal support in the form of an elastic binder, belt or corset."[10] The Suckley diary is dotted with references to back pain. After Bremerton he never stood up for more than a few excruciating minutes at a time.

On August 18, Franklin met at the White House with Harry Truman. "Dad was appalled by Mr. Roosevelt's medical condition," Truman's daughter Margaret later wrote. "The President had just returned from a Pacific inspection trip. It had been an exhausting ordeal for him and he suffered, as we know, at least one cardiac seizure during the journey to Bremerton.[11] He spoke with difficulty. 'It doesn't seem to be any mental lapse of any kind, but physically he's just going to pieces,' Dad said. 'I'm very much concerned about him.' The President alluded only once, and then obliquely, to the seriousness of his condition. He asked Dad how he planned to campaign, and Dad said he was thinking of using an airplane. The President vetoed the idea, saying, 'One of us has to stay alive.'"[12]

The next evening Franklin left Washington for Hyde Park. "The P. had a good color & everyone thinks him looking well," Daisy Suckley wrote on August 20. "He does, except for a sort of pallor and a strained look about the mouth which you see in sick people ... He says he feels pretty well, but tired most of the time. He has to save his strength to appear a few times in public before the election," she continued. "He spoke from the destroyer in Bremerton standing

---

8 Rosenman, 462.

9 The complete speech can be seen at https://www.youtube.com/watch?v= 0xL0pscCMKw&t=1122s.

10 Ferrell, 69.

11 This refers to the attack of "angina" while speaking at Bremerton alleged to have occurred by Howard Bruenn. It also reveals that both Truman and his daughter bought into Bruenn's story.

12 "Daughter Tells How Truman Got Word of FDR's Death." *The Evening News*, Newburgh, NY, December 7, 1972.

up for the first time in a year, & found it pretty exhausting. He said the muscles are 'just not there.'"[13]

Observations of unremitting fatigue and accelerated physical decline dot the Suckley diary during this period:

August 29: The Pres. appeared quite late for cocktails and dinner, looking awfully tired. He has lost 2 ½ lb. since starting on the trip to Hawaii & they are giving him an eggnog at 11 and a large glass of orange juice at 4, plus his regular meals.

September 4: The Pres was feeling 'low' and 'logy.' He didn't know what was the matter with him.

September 6: At 4 p.m. the Pres. telephoned from Wash. said he felt miserable—'like a boiled owl'—his voice sounded heavy—he said it was a stomach upset ... I was much worried and called him at 9:30. He was in bed, had had milk toast & would soon go to sleep—He sounded better & thought he had just eaten something that disagreed.

September 10: His back is not so straight as it was—he is tired, and sitting upright is an effort. [a strong suggestion of a spinal problem].

I went up and kissed him—he said he had had four awful days and was really tired. When asked how he was feeling, he said he felt just tired, not up to anything and that, like on the trip to [South America] in 1936, he couldn't sign his name properly.

September 11: The Pres. worries me. He gets so awfully tired and has no chance to rest ... He is to speak at the Teamsters' Union dinner at The Statler, Sat. the 23rd. He said, 'I just can't stand up to make that speech.'"

On September 12, Lahey was blindsided by a newspaperman who came to Boston to ask if he had treated the president. Lahey refused to answer and fired off a letter to McIntire to cover his tracks. "I told him that I did not see how an editor could send an assistant editor on such a foolish mission. He asked me if I had seen the president professionally and I told him that is something he had no right to ask and that the only answer I could make was that you had told me, and it was my opinion, that he was now in excellent health." [14]

---

13 *Suckley Diary.*
14 Lahey to McIntire, McIntire papers, FDRL.

Reelection was not a sure thing. GOP jibes about "tired old men" running the government was having an effect. Democrats were leading in the polls, but not by the comfortable margin they enjoyed in 1936 or 1940. But Franklin was able to summon the inner strength to ensure victory—thanks to his performances at two events.

He was to speak on September 23 at a dinner hosted by the International Brotherhood of Teamsters at the Washington Statler Hotel. A supportive audience offered a chance to show that his hapless showing at Bremerton had been an aberration. Sam Rosenman and Frances Perkins drafted a pro-labor text, but days before the dinner Dewey gave a speech essentially endorsing the Democrat's labor record. Perkins retooled the draft, but Franklin told her not to worry. "I'm not going to use any of the stuff you sent me," he said. "I've got my mind on something else, and I'm going to have a good time."[15]

He certainly did. Speaking from his chair on the dais, Franklin touched only briefly on labor matters. Instead he used the occasion to defend his record, needle Dewey and his recent speech as "the Old Guard trying to pass itself off as the New Deal," and lambaste Republican falsehoods. "These Republican leaders have not been content with attacks on me, or my wife, or on my sons. No, not content with that, they now include my little dog, Fala," Franklin told his audience. "Well, of course, I don't resent attacks, and my family doesn't resent attacks, but Fala *does* resent them. You know, Fala is Scotch, and being a Scottie, as soon as he learned that the Republican fiction writers—in Congress and out—had concocted a story that I had left him behind on the Aleutian Islands and had sent a destroyer back to find him—at a cost to the taxpayers of two or three, or eight or twenty million dollars—his Scotch soul was furious! He has not been the same dog since. I am accustomed to hearing malicious falsehoods about myself, such as that old, worm-eaten chestnut that I have represented myself as indispensable (chuckling). But I think I have a right to resent, to object, to libelous statements about my dog!"[16,17]

The audience roared with laughter, as did millions listening on the radio. "No one could have delivered this short passage more effectively," Rosenman wrote. "His mock-serious face and his sad tone of voice set the audience shouting

---

15 Perkins, 114.
16 *New York Times*, September 24, 1944.
17 https://www.youtube.com/watch?v=b9ImwBG8ods.

WAR MANPOWER COMMISSION

WASHINGTON, D. C., 25

PROCUREMENT and ASSIGNMENT SERVICE for
PHYSICIANS, DENTISTS and VETERINARIANS

September 12, 1944

Vice Admiral Ross T. McIntire
Surgeon General of the Navy
Washington, D. C.

Dear Admiral McIntire:

I have to write you this letter to protect myself against
any possible mis-statement that may be made. A Mr. Charles
Ross of the St. Louis Despatch telephoned me that his editor,
Mr. Pulitzer, had commissioned him to come to Boston and see
me about something of a confidential nature which he could
not discuss over the telephone. I told him that it was a
long trip for him to make on such a vague basis, that I would
see him here, and I saw him this morning.

He stated that he had been confidentially committed to run
down a rumor that following the collapse of Germany the
President would resign in order to handle a peace settlement. He asked me if I had discussed any such thing with
the President or if he had given me any such information.
I told him how ridiculous this was and that the only time
I saw the President was when I got in trouble with the
Procurement and Assignment Service, and that he had never
made a remark to me which had any political implication.

I told him that I did not see how an editor could send an
assistant editor on such a foolish mission. He asked me if
I had seen the President professionally and I told him that
that was something that I felt he had no right to ask, and
that the only answer I could make was that you had told me,
and it was my opinion, that he was now in excellent health.

If all of the above seems foolish, it is merely to state the
facts lest there be any distortion at any time. I suppose we
must expect more and more of this business as we get nearer
to election time.

With kindest personal regards, I am

Sincerely yours,

Frank H. Lahey, M. D.
Chairman, Directing Board

*Apologetic letter from Dr. Frank Lahey to Ross
McIntire, September 12, 1944.*

with glee, but he continued through the statement with the same serious note of righteous indignation, never cracking a smile until the end."[18]

Franklin's bravura performance was one of the most effective campaign speeches any American candidate ever gave and went a long way to reassure voters their president was up to the task of running the country for another four years.

Though Franklin had proved he could rally, Daisy Suckley wrote that he must have delivered the speech "through sheer will power & determination."[19] He was still a very sick man, and it was showing. A week earlier, he had been in Quebec to meet with Churchill and Canadian Prime Minister Mackenzie King. "It seemed to me ... that he had failed very much since I last saw him," King wrote. "He is very much thinner in body and also is much thinner in his face. He looks distinctly older and worn. I confess I was just a little shocked at his appearance ... As Roosevelt was speaking the language was very loosely used ... he had lost his old hearty self and his laugh. Conceded he has suffered a great deal and really is a man who is gradually losing his strength ... He certainly has not the grasp today that he had a year ago."[20] Franklin's naval aide, Admiral Wilson Brown, told King that Ross McIntire was "really concerned about him." After Franklin departed, King noticed the absence of an American flag outside the assembly building and felt it was "an ill omen, as if the President might be the first to be taken of the three of us."[21,22] Churchill's physician, Lord Moran, also sensed grave problems in Quebec. "Roosevelt's health impaired his judgment and sapped his resolve to get to the bottom of each problem." And, possibly alluding to the effect of malignancy, added "Men at this time of life do not go thin all of a sudden just for nothing."[23]

The after-dinner entertainment on September 15 was the biopic *Wilson*, featuring an Oscar nominated performance by Alexander Knox in the title role. As Franklin was watching the scene portraying the former president's disability after his stroke, something he had witnessed, he was observed by Howard

---

18 Rosenman, 477.
19 *Suckley Diary*, September 25, 1944.
20 Ferrell, 85.
21 *Mackenzie King Diary*, September 10–11 as quoted in Ferrell, footnote 30, 163.
22 Ferrell, 85.
23 Charles McMoran Wilson (Lord Moran), Churchill: The Diaries of Lord Moran: the Struggle for Survival, 1940–1965. Boston: Houghton Mifflin, 1966, 192.

Bruenn to become visibly distressed. "By God, that's not going to happen to me!" Franklin, muttered, as his blood pressure soared to 240/130.[24]

Franklin was asked about his health only once during the presidential campaign—at a press conference on October 17. "Mr. President, have you read the ominous reports about your health, printed by some of the more rugged correspondents?" a reporter asked sarcastically. Franklin joined the laughter that greeted the question. "More *what* correspondents?" he replied. "Look—don't get me commenting on the word 'rugged,' because I might say things that I would be sorry for. On some of them, I think I know more about their health than they know about mine. I think it's pretty good health."[25]

Joseph P. Kennedy met with Franklin at the White House on October 26. "If I hadn't been warned by the stories of his illness ... I would have been shocked beyond words," Kennedy wrote to his daughter Kathleen. "He sat behind his desk, and his face was as gray as his hair ... During the entire conversation, I was convinced that he is far from a well man. He is thin; he has an unhealthy color. His hands shake violently when he tries to take a drink of water. About 10 per cent of the time that he is talking, his words are not clearly enunciated."[26]

Kennedy also recounted a story told him by former Supreme Court Justice James "Jimmy" Byrnes.[27] On October 16, the justices had visited Franklin. He was in such bad shape that Justice Owen Roberts told Byrnes, "I think this is cruel. This man is in no shape to talk, and we should get him out."

Kennedy described meetings with Democratic Party chairman Robert Hannegan and with Franklin's running mate Harry Truman—both of whom said they didn't expect him to live long. "And if I haven't made it strong enough before I state again," he told his daughter, "both Truman and Hannegan discussed what they would do when the President died."[28] Truman was later quoted by his assistant, Daniel Noyes, as saying that after the July 1944 Democratic convention, "I watched him very carefully, and from that point on I was worried to death each time I saw him ... I wake up every morning in a cold sweat dreading that it might be the last day."[29]

---

24 Ferrell, 85.
25 Press conferences of FDR, October 17, 1944.
26 Smith, A., ed. *Hostage to Fortune: The Letters of Joseph P. Kennedy.* Viking Press, 2001, 607.
27 *Ibid.*, 612; FDR Day by Day, October 16, 1944.
28 Smith, A., 612.
29 Evans, H.E., *The Hidden Campaign: FDR's Health and the 1944 Election.* Routledge, 2002, 111.

Most newspaper columnists and editorial writers refrained from commenting on the president's health, but not the leaders of the anti-Roosevelt press. The New York *Daily News* and its sister paper, the *Chicago Tribune*, published editorials predicting Franklin would die in office. "Evidence increases that Mr. Roosevelt is not in fit physical condition to meet those demands," the *Tribune* wrote on October 17. "If he dies or becomes incapacitated, [those around him] figure they can do business with Truman."[30] A week before the election, the *Tribune* dropped all pretense: "In view of Mr. Roosevelt's age and brittle health, a vote for Mr. Roosevelt is very likely to be a vote for Truman for President."[31]

As in 1936, when he banned photographs "when [Franklin] is unaware,"[32] Steve Early went to work to enhance Franklin's visual image. "For many months, photographers have revealed deepening lines of age and weariness in the president's face," the Syracuse *Post-Standard* reported. "Now, orders have been given that there must be no more pictures taken in the telltale glare of flash bulbs and unflattering floodlights. [Movie producer] Walter Wanger sent expert electricians from Hollywood to supervise lighting of future Roosevelt pictures, the first of which, taken two nights ago, made the president look much younger and healthier. Such precautions are an indication of the anxiety felt in White House circles over the president's health."[33] Wanger likely also dispatched professional makeup artists.

The Fala speech had reassured voters about Franklin's mental acuity, but not his physical stamina. Although the White House had declared the president would give no more public campaign speeches, Bob Hannegan persuaded Franklin's aides they needed to demonstrate more conclusively that he was physically up to the job. The team organized a four-hour swing through New York City for October 21, including a speech at Ebbets Field, home of the Brooklyn Dodgers. "After the people have seen him," Hannegan said, "they can make up their own minds about his vigor and health."[34]

The planners couldn't have picked a worse day. "It had never rained more incessantly and gloomily than now, and what had been a steady, lashing rain

---

30 "The President's Health." *Chicago Tribune*, October 17, 1944.
31 "A Vote for FDR May Be a Vote for Truman." *Chicago Tribune*, October 28, 1944.
32 "Roosevelt Bars Photos Catching Him Unaware." *New York Times*, February 3, 1936.
33 *Syracuse Post-Standard*, undated (late October 1944), Stephen T. Early scrapbooks, FDRL.
34 *Time*, October 29, 1944.

in Brooklyn turned into a torrent in Manhattan," wrote *Time*.[35] For fifty-one miles, Franklin braved the elements in the back seat of an open Packard, waving his hat to the crowd. Photos showed his trademark pince-nez glasses spattered with rain. Moreover, it was cold. A crowd of between 1.5 and 3 million along the motorcade route stood for hours, "their legs chilled by the wind" and "their teeth chattering," *The New York Times* wrote.[36]

At several points "the President's car was turned out of the parade into the warmth of a heated [garage]. Secret Service agents quickly lifted the President from the car and stretched him out full length on blankets laid on the floor," biographer Hugh Gallagher wrote. "They removed his clothes down to the skin. He was toweled dry and given a rubdown. He was redressed in dry clothes, brandy was poured down his throat, and he was lifted back into the car. The pit stop was quickly done, and the President was soon back in the cavalcade."[37]

Franklin capped the day with an uninspired speech to the Foreign Policy Association at the Waldorf Astoria Hotel. Members of the press noticed he was slurring his words. *Newsweek* reported the speech was a "fighting message delivered in a non-fighting fashion."[38] McIntire claimed a "loose bridge" had made the president sound "like he was lisping."[39] The real "problem" with Franklin's speech was likely nothing more than a simple case of alcohol intoxication. As Grace Tully noted, "After the tour and before the speech Roosevelt followed McIntire's prescription for 'a couple of hookers' of medicinal bourbon whisky, a nap, and another medicinal treatment, and then attended a cocktail party and drank martinis." [40] Franklin held his alcohol well, but likely resorted to using it as an anesthetic to ease his severe pain. After the dinner, Franklin began his journey to Hyde Park by simply taking an elevator down to Grand Central Station Track 61, located in the basement of the hotel, where his private railway car, *Ferdinand Magellan*, was waiting. The escape route had been constructed by Vincent Astor when he built the hotel in 1929.[41]

35 *Ibid.*
36 *New York Times*, October 22, 1944.
37 Gallagher, 195.
38 *Newsweek*, October 30, 1944, 43–44.
39 Gunther, J. *Roosevelt in Retrospect.* New York: Harper & Brothers, 1950, 28.
40 Tully, 281.
41 There is a lot of mythology connected to Track 61. The most comprehensive article about it can be found at https://gothamist.com/arts-entertainment/a-look-inside-track-61-the-secret-train-platform-under-the-waldorf-astoria (last accessed March 18, 2022).

Franklin was so invigorated by the reception to his madcap day of campaigning—and the positive response from the press, which declared that he had put the health issue to rest—that he scheduled repeat performances in Philadelphia, Chicago, and Boston, the last more probably an excuse to sneak in an examination by Frank Lahey.[42] "Now fired with the old fire-horse enthusiasm," wrote *Time*, "Candidate Roosevelt would give it all he had."[43] Franklin was voted into office for an unprecedented fourth term on November 7. The Fala Speech and the multi-city tours were successful beyond their wildest dreams. An editorial in the *New York Post* on October 30 glowed:

> "We marvel that the President has not contented himself with the work he has already done. For most great men that would be all that mind and body and spirit could carry. We marvel also that some fail to grasp or refuse to understand the dynamic quality of his leadership, that they do not examine him against the demands that will be made upon us as a democracy today and tomorrow. Indeed, some, like the *Herald Tribune*, propose that he be examined physically by 'impartial experts.' The *Tribune* says the question is not whether the President will live four years longer, but whether he is still strong enough for his job. The Republicans are now campaigning with a stethoscope. They are doing this because they dare not test their candidate, in the closing week of the campaign, by any other standard than his age. What More? The President has aged. Most men do at 62. He has lost some weight. But no 'impartial experts' are required to determine that a man of the President's years, who can ride in open cars for hours through wind, rain and snow and deliver three major addresses within eight days in New York, Philadelphia and Chicago, is a good deal stronger than most of us. We would like to ask the *Tribune*: Is the President functioning effectively today? Is there anything in his performance of the past ten days that shows him tired or weak in mind or body? Is there any other voice in the world today which presents the principles of foreign policy to which the *Tribune* itself has long been committed? The President during the past ten days has unfolded, with intellectual precision and vigor unsurpassed at any point in his career, his program for leading America along the road to peace, security and freedom. A man ill in body or tired in mind could not have done what we all have just seen and heard him do. A man who has grown older, but who is strong still and has lost none of the fire of his faith, could and did do it. So we wonder when, in the opinion of the *Tribune*, the President might prove unable to carry out tasks as great as those he has just performed publicly. Next

---

42 The warmup speech at Fenway Park was given by Orson Welles. Frank Sinatra sang "America the Beautiful" See: https://www.wellesnet.com/fdr-orson-welles-frank-sinatra/. No film of the event survives.

43 *Time*, October 29, 1944.

week? Next year? Or after four more vigorous years? The *Tribune* is encouraging speculation that is both futile and dangerous for the country. The real test is which of the candidates, as of Election Day, has proved himself better able to lead us during the next four years."

Ross McIntire himself could not have written a more positive testimonial.

Franklin's popular vote margin was comfortable but by no means overwhelming—53 to 46 percent, though he scored his customary landslide in the Electoral College, besting Dewey by 432 votes to 99. Ten days after the election, Rev. Endicott Peabody died at age 87. In 1937, Franklin had designated him to officiate at his funeral.

There had not been any significant leak about Franklin's cancers until December 14, when J. Edgar Hoover notified Early he'd received word of "another avalanche of rumors in and around Washington."[44] The memorandum revealed information bureau agents had discovered that went far beyond presidential heart problems, including plans for an operation for prostate cancer after the election.[45]

The memorandum rings of truth. Franklin was indeed in Warm Springs between November 27 and December 18, 1944. Hoover named two doctors, Frank Lahey and William Calhoun Stirling [misspelled "Sterling" in the document], who knew about Roosevelt's cancer and had never been publicly identified as having treated the president. Numerous credible accounts uncovered by Harry Goldsmith describe Dr. Lahey as being forthcoming about the services he provided the president, including the fact that a malignancy was involved.

Lahey's insistence to treat prominent patients at his Boston clinic is also well established. In 1953 Lahey's deputy, Dr. Richard Cattell, repaired British Foreign Secretary Anthony Eden's bile duct after London surgeons had botched the job. At Lahey's insistence the Eden repair surgery took place in Boston over heated objections from Prime Minister Winston Churchill.[46,47]

---

44 J. Edgar Hoover to Stephen Early, December 14, 1944, FBI.
45 FBI Memorandum, courtesy of Margheritta Stirling Allardice.
46 *Time*, June 15, 1953.
47 Harry Goldsmith devoted an entire chapter of his book to Franklin's prostate cancer. A very strong circumstantial case is presented. The entire story is far too convoluted for this book and many of the details are quoted in the text. See: Goldsmith, H.A., *Conspiracy of Silence*. New York: Stratton Press (2nd edition), 2019, 124–144.

December 14, 1944

MEMORANDUM

Recurrent rumors concerning the President's health are surging and echoing through Washington. The present "inside" story currently being discussed by most people, but mostly newspapermen, is alleged to emanate from "informed White House circles." The story is as follows:

Dr. William Calhoun "Pete" Sterling has established a good reputatic for his surgery specializing in prostate, kidney and similar ailments. The story states that "Pete" Sterling was recently called for an extensi examination of the President and although an operation was necessary, Dr. Sterling refused to operate because of the very bad condition of the President's health. "Pete" Sterling is alleged to have declined to operate on the grounds that the President's condition was so bad that he would probably die from the operation and Dr. Sterling did not want t jeopardize his entire future in the medical practice by being known as the man who had killed the President. Accordingly, the "White House" called into the case Dr. Frank Lahey of Boston. Dr. Lahey allegedly concluded that an operation was absolutely necessary and "the White Hous decided that the operation would be performed after the Presidential election.

The story continues that the President is suffering from "proxysmal tachycorida" (phonetic), which is described as a sudden increase in hea action which causes trembling, shaking, etc. This affliction, it is stated, frequently follows polio attacks. The rumor then outlines that Dr. Lahey was insistent that the President build up his physical condition, as a result of which the President went to Warm Springs, Georgia, for a stay of ten days, which has been lengthened to 20 days, in order build up all possible resistance. Dr. Lahey allegedly has demanded tha the operation be performed at the Lahey Clinic in Boston because it is alleged Lahey feels that the advertising value of his operating upon th President in Boston will be "worth millions of dollars to the Lahey Clinic." Dr. Lahey is supposed to reason that even though the operatic is unsuccessful and the President dies, most people would concede that Dr. Lahey and his Clinic must be preeminent if the President went there for an operation. Accordingly, it is alleged that the rumor has spread throughout New England that the President is to be operated upon in Boston, the operation to take place about the first of the year or possibly even sooner.

The rumor states that Dr. Lahey performs many of his operations at the Baptist Hospital in Boston and that on or about December 8th a Unit States Secret Service man from Washington, whose name is Barker, was in Boston checking upon the facilities, etc. at the Baptist Hospital in Boston.

62-76894-17

FBI memorandum, December 9, 1944. Courtesy Herbert Hoover Library and Museum, West Branch, Iowa.

The December 1944 FBI memo also hinted that Stirling had been one of the sources. The loose-lipped urologist gave similar information to Walter Trohan. He was also the likely source for the 1941 *Abwehr* report about Franklin's health.

Lahey's business manager, confidante, and executor, Linda Strand, told Goldsmith that "she had met FDR at the New England Baptist Hospital on several occasions, where he had been admitted under a different name."[48] Stanley P. Lovell, longtime director of research and development for the Office of Strategic Services (OSS), wrote in his memoir that, at about the time of the 1944 Democratic National Convention, "we in OSS ... had seen a report from the Lahey Clinic in Boston whose doctors, after examining the president, stated that he would not survive another term."[49]

Goldsmith revealed in 2005 that, at the very least, an examination of Franklin took place at Baptist Hospital in Boston. Franklin's "day by day" calendar records a gap of time on November 4, 1944, sufficient for him to have visited Lahey prior to speaking at Fenway Park at 9 that evening.[50]

To the contrary, there was not enough time for Franklin to recover from the surgery mentioned in the FBI memo in the ten weeks between Election Day and his inauguration on January 20, 1945. On January 30, with Franklin on his way to Yalta, Hollywood celebrities including actress Veronica Lake attended the annual charity "birthday ball" at the White House for the benefit of the March of Dimes.[51] Unsolicited, Eleanor pulled Lake aside and told the actress that upon her husband's return he was planning to undergo surgery for

---

48 Goldsmith, 170.

49 Lovell, S.P., *Of Spies and Stratagems.* New York: Permabooks, 1964, 70.

50 In a long endnote in *The Dying President*, 158, Robert Ferrell relates a credible account of Doctor Samuel Day's meeting with Dr. George Pack where he related a story told to him by Lahey "that President Roosevelt and his entourage came to Boston by special train to see Dr. Lahey prior to his final race for reelection in 1944.... It was found that he had advanced cancer of the stomach." The story melds a number of unrelated facts together but the train trip described was probably the one where FDR also spoke at Fenway Park.

51 The March of Dimes was initiated in 1938 as an extension of FDR's National Foundation for Infantile Paralysis. The name was coined by entertainer Eddie Cantor to be reminiscent of the popular newsreel series the "March of Time." The charity funded Jonas Salk's development of a polio vaccine, which was announced on April 12, 1945, the tenth anniversary of FDR's death. The charity's success is unique. To date it is the only one which found a cure for the disease for which it was created!

cancer of the prostate.[52,53] By the time Franklin returned, he was far too sick to undergo such an operation and he had his sights set to be in San Francisco on April 25.

52 Veronica Lake and Donald Bain, *Veronica*. New York: Citadel Press, 1970, 132.
53 Lake was at the White House with a group of Hollywood celebrities for Franklin's annual Birthday Ball to raise funds for polio research and treatment.

■ Chapter 23
■ "He'll Come Out of It. He Always Does."

Franklin Delano Roosevelt was epileptic for the last seventeen months of his life.[1] He had frequent sudden spells of inattentiveness, staring blankly and dropping his jaw, then just as quickly snapping back into focus.

From Alexander the Great to Charles Dickens, numerous historical figures have been epileptic. Eleanor Roosevelt's uncle President Theodore Roosevelt is purported to have been stricken as a child. Her father, Elliott—Theodore's brother—died at age 34 shortly after a seizure related to his chronic alcoholism.

The brain functions by creating electrical impulses and communicating them along nerves. Seizures are bursts of abnormal electricity that overcome that function. Epilepsy is simply defined today as more than one seizure. It had been described for eons but its cause did not begin to be explained until English neurologist John Hughlings Jackson discovered in the 1880s that the violent convulsive spasms that march across the body arose from specific areas of the brain. Another pioneer was Englishman William Gowers, whose classic 1907 textbook, *The Borderland of Epilepsy*, raised awareness of seizures as the cause of a wide variety of neurologic symptoms.

The first effective treatment for seizures dates back to 1857, when potassium bromide was introduced by Sir Charles Locock, an obstetrician to Queen Victoria.[2] That substance had severe side effects and was abandoned after the debut in 1912 of phenobarbital (Luminal), a remarkably safe and effective compound still in use today. Howard Bruenn admitted prescribing phenobarbital for Franklin in 1944 but only as "a brake on excessive activity as well as a cushion against possible emotional trauma."[3] The only other anticonvulsant in use during Franklin's lifetime was phenytoin (Dilantin), introduced by American neurologists H. Houston Merritt and Tracy J. Putnam in 1938. Dilantin remained a staple of epilepsy treatment into the twenty-first century. It is logical to assume Franklin was treated with Dilantin, but no evidence has

---

1 Epilepsy is simply defined as having more than one seizure, no matter what the type.
2 There is no evidence Locock used the drug on the Queen, nor that she was epileptic.
3 Ferrell, 69.

surfaced.[4] Franklin's neurological care in the 1940s was most probably overseen by Winchell McKendree Craig, chairman of neurosurgery at the National Naval Medical Center at Bethesda, Maryland.[5]

The relationship of seizures to abnormal brain waves came to be understood in 1941 with the advent of electroencephalography (EEG). American neurologist Frederick Gibbs developed EEG based on research by a German psychiatrist, Hans Berger. The National Naval Medical Center began using EEG soon after it was discovered. It is reasonable to assume that Franklin's seizures were diagnosed and treated there.[6,7] The American military, especially the Navy, has always been at the cutting edge of medical innovation.

Epilepsy is more than just violent grand mal convulsions. The disease reveals itself in many ways—a subtle blink, the twitch of a hand, a smell of burnt rubber, or, in Franklin's case, a staring spell and a sagging jaw. Even today, onlookers often misinterpret the signs of epilepsy. This explains the confusion about Franklin's neurological symptoms, as even doctors did not recognize many of these signs as manifestations of epilepsy until the second half of the twentieth century.

Frances Perkins gave one of the most graphic descriptions of Franklin's seizures. "The change in his appearance had to do with the oncoming of a kind of glassy eye and an extremely drawn look around the eyes and cheeks and even a sort of dropping of the muscles of the jaws and mouth as though they weren't working exactly," Perkins told Columbia University historians in 1955. "I think they were but there was a great weakness in those muscles. Also, if you saw him close, you would see that his hands were weak. When he fainted as he did occasionally—not for many years but for several years that was all

---

4 Merritt was Chief of Neurology at Columbia at the time when Anna's third husband, internist James Halsted, was an attending physician there.

5 Craig held a similar position at Mayo Clinic before the war. An interview between the author and his nephew living in Seattle confirmed the relationship between FDR and his "Uncle Wink."

6 "Oh, My Aching Head Interpreted by E.E.G." *National Naval Medical Center News*, volume 1, number 3, Bethesda, MD, January 20, 1945, 3.

7 Until the mid-1970s, imaging of the brain and spinal cord was limited to angiography, the injection of radiopaque contrast material into blood vessels, and a few primitive, painful, and invasive radiological procedures—pneumoencephalography (replacing the spinal fluid with air to provide X-ray contrast of intracranial contents) (reference to FDR having a pneumoencephalogram) and myelography (introducing iodine-based radiopaque contrast material into the spinal canal).

accentuated. It would be momentary. It would be very brief and he'd be back again."[8]

Anna Roosevelt's third husband, Dr. James Halsted, wrote to Howard Bruenn that his wife "does remember times when [Franklin] seemed very quiet, almost introspective, starting in December 1943."[9] Anna herself recollected these episodes far more graphically to a close friend, urologist Dr. Louis E. Schmidt. In 1948, Schmidt paraphrased Anna's remarks to *Chicago Tribune* reporter, Orville "Doc" Dwyer.

"The doctor told me that from what Anna has outlined to him Franklin D. Roosevelt was for a long time before he died—and particularly when he went to Yalta and Tehran—suffering from hemorrhages of the brain," Dwyer reported. "The doctor said he died 'from a big hemorrhage' but for several years before his death had a lot of 'little hemorrhages,' small blood vessels bursting in his brain. When these burstings occurred—and they were frequent during his last years—he could be unconscious (completely out) although sitting up and apparently functioning for periods of from a few seconds to several minutes. Dr. Schmidt said he has no doubt from his conversations with Anna that they were occurring regularly at the time he was meeting with Churchill and Stalin and holding other momentous conferences of the utmost importance to the United States. He said the effect would be that he would be cognizant of what was going on, then suddenly lose the thread completely for anywhere from a few seconds to two or three minutes—and that he could not possibly have known what was going on in between."[10] Similarly, Anna also told publisher of the *Chicago Tribune*, "Colonel Robert McCormick in 1947, 'FDR was sick for months before he ran for a third [actually the fourth] time—his mind drifted—amnesia—that when talked to he would forget what was being said and come back into the conversation not knowing what was said.'"[11]

The "burstings" and "amnesia" Anna described are classified today as "complex partial" or "absence" seizures—episodes of loss of consciousness without

---

8 Oral History of Frances Perkins. *Columbia University Libraries Oral History Office, Notable New Yorkers*, 1955, Part 8, Session 12, 283–284 http://www.columbia.edu/cu/lweb/digital/collections/nny/perkinsf/index.html (last accessed March 4, 2019).
9 Howard Bruenn papers, FDR Library.
10 Memorandum of Orville Dwyer, *Walter Trohan Papers*, Herbert Hoover Library, North Branch, IA.
11 Memo of P. Maloney to Walter Trohan, August 1, 1947, Trohan Papers, Herbert Hoover Library, North Branch, IA.

convulsive movements.[12] This largely explains why Dr. Karl Wold misdiagnosed Franklin's seizures as "small strokes" in his 1949 *Look* magazine article. A chapter in a 1986 book by neurosurgeon Burt Edward Park about Franklin's health, *The Impact of Illness on World Leaders*, devotes considerable discussion to multiple transient lapses of consciousness. Park labeled them "transient encephalopathy," but they were undoubtedly seizures.

New York Times reporter Turner Catledge described such an episode occurring during a meeting with Franklin in July 1944. "When I entered the president's office, I had my first glimpse of him in several months," Catledge wrote decades later. "I was shocked and horrified—so much of my impulse was to turn around and leave. I felt I was seeing something I shouldn't see. He had lost a great deal of weight. His shirt collar hung so loose around his neck that you could have put your hand inside it. He was sitting there with a vague glassy-eyed expression on his face and his mouth hanging open. Reluctantly, I sat down and we started talking. I expected him to ask me about the political situation, but he never did. He would start talking about something, then in mid-sentence he would stop and his mouth would drop open and he'd sit staring at me in silence. I knew he was a terribly sick man ... And my talk lasted more than an hour with him. ... Repeatedly he would lose his train of thought, stop, and stare blankly at me. It was an agonizing experience for me. Finally a waiter brought his lunch, and [Pa] Watson said his luncheon guest was waiting, and I was able to make my escape."[13]

Catledge had happened upon a legitimate and powerful news story—visible firsthand evidence of Franklin's ill health, rumors of which already were sweeping Washington. He opted not to tell the story until publishing his memoirs more than a quarter century after Franklin's death.

Howard Bruenn denied anything unusual occurred during Franklin's trip to Hawaii, but in August 1944, a "high-ranking officer" described a seizure to Roosevelt critic John D. Flynn.

"For the first time we hear of his conversation falling into intervals of irrelevance," said the officer, "Here at a dinner he sat reading a short speech. Suddenly he faltered and paused, his eyes became glassy, consciousness drifted from him. The man at his side nudged him, shook him a little, pointed at the place in the manuscript at which [Franklin] broke off and said 'Here, Mr. President, is

---

12 They are often confused with "petit mal," seizures which only occur in children.
13 Catledge, T., *My Life and the Times*. New York: Harper and Row, 1971, 146.

your place.' With an effort he resumed. As he was wheeled from his quarters, officers noticed his head drooping forward, his jaw hanging loosely."[14]

White House butler Alonzo Fields described Franklin's seizures in a 1994 episode of the PBS documentary series *American Experience*. "You could see him just fade away," Fields recalled. "He would come to the table sometimes and he would be bright and cheerful, but if any agitation happened in the conversation, he would again sag and he'd sort of droop and drop his head or he would drop his jaw." In the same film, former Secret Service agent Milton Lipson recalled, "several occasions when he had the misfortune to fall out of his chair and you'd have to come in and there was the President of the United States helpless on the floor, and you gently pick him up, say nothing about it, put him back on the chair and that was it. But your heart would break."

The best testimony to the frequency of Franklin's seizures comes from a description of a White House visit by Senator Francis Maloney (D-Connecticut) in January 1945. As related to historian Doris Kearns Goodwin, "Maloney went in and sat down. Roosevelt looked up but said nothing, his eyes fixed in a strange stare. After a few moments of silence, Maloney realized that Roosevelt had absolutely no idea who his visitor was," wrote Goodwin. "A pious Catholic, Maloney crossed himself and ran to get 'Pa' Watson, fearing the president had suffered a stroke. 'Don't worry,' Watson said. 'He'll come out of it. He always does.' By the time Maloney returned to the Oval Office, Roosevelt had pulled himself together. Smiling broadly, he greeted Maloney warmly and launched into a spirited conversation."[15]

Despite the frequency of these events in the last seventeen months of Franklin's life, it is notable that three of the people who were with him the most, Howard Bruenn, Daisy Suckley, and Eleanor, never reported them. They all had surely witnessed countless events, yet they remained silent.

Franklin's seizures were first described in *FDR's Deadly Secret* in 2010. In 2011, the American Academy of Neurology validated the diagnosis with the publication of *The Epilepsy of Franklin Delano Roosevelt* in its preeminent peer-reviewed journal.[16]

---

14 Flynn, J.T., *The Roosevelt Myth*. Garden City, 1948, 403.
15 Goodwin, 501. Goodwin identifies the noted economist Eliot Janeway as her source.
16 Lomazow, S. "The Epilepsy of Franklin Delano Roosevelt." *Neurology* February 15, 2011, 76(7). See: https://n.neurology.org/content/76/7/668.

■ Chapter 24
■ Race Against Death

By the end of 1944, many of Franklin's physical pleasures were being denied him. His afternoon swim was forbidden. From as many as forty cigarettes a day, he was down to about six. His diet was more therapeutic than pleasurable. When he deviated from it he paid the price of severe abdominal pain. His hands refused to function. They had been shaky for a year, but he was now unable to hold a cup and saucer steadily or even light his own cigarette. His immaculate penmanship had degenerated into a tragic scrawl.

Intimates who had shared his earlier triumphs—his mother, Louis Howe, Missy LeHand, and Harry Hopkins, were dead or dying. Franklin's private life had long since taken a separate path from Eleanor's. His sons were all away at war. "Nowhere in the world really was there anyone for him with whom he could unlock his mind and his thoughts," James wrote. "Politics, domestic economy, war strategy, postwar planning he could talk over with dozens of persons. Of what was inside him, Father talked to no one."[1] Unbeknownst to James though, his sister Anna and, even more so Daisy Suckley, were consistent sources of comfort. A lesser man would have given up, but Franklin was determined to achieve his most important goal—the establishment of the United Nations. As his health worsened, his efforts became more urgent.

On November 27, Franklin announced the resignation of Cordell Hull as secretary of state.[2] Four hours later, he boarded a train for Warm Springs, where he hoped to regain the strength and agility needed to stand and deliver his inaugural address on January 20. His weight was down to 160 pounds. "He looked pale & thin & tired," Daisy Suckley wrote on November 28. "He looks ten years older than last year, to me—Of course I wouldn't confess that to anyone, last of all to him, but he knows it himself."[3]

Infections, heart failure, cancer, epilepsy, and the side effects of the medicines used to treat them were making it difficult for Franklin to stay awake—and

---

1 Roosevelt and Shalett, 317.
2 Hull was widely rumored to have tuberculosis but more likely had a similarly pathological noninfectious condition, Sarcoidosis.
3 *Suckley Diary*, November 29, 1944.

when he was, to maintain his train of thought. "The Pres. Finally came out of his room at about 12:30 and ... seemed tired and listless, didn't talk as much as usual," Daisy wrote on December 1. "He ate a pretty good lunch, however— Afterwards, he went to his room for an hour of sleep."

The next day, Daisy found Franklin feeling cold, sitting up in bed with a sweater on. However, "he feels more chipper this morning, after a good night's sleep, *though the back still bothers him somewhat*," she wrote (emphasis added).[4] On December 5, she noted, "He needs rest & rest & rest, interspersed with fresh air & cheerful conversation."

On December 7, Franklin decided to go for a swim—against doctor's orders. "[A longtime patient] was in the pool when we got there. It was warm in the enclosed pool, but the water temperature was only about 89, instead of the 93–94 it is where it comes out of the ground," Daisy wrote. "Dr. Bruenn wanted F. to be in the water at the most 10 minutes—But F. got talking about old times & then about his muscles; he tried to walk & discovered his hips are stiff, and unless he loosens them up he will not be able to stand for his inauguration. So now there is a new problem of loosening the President's hips! He thinks he can do it by lying flat on a board, with his legs hanging, to stretch the front hip muscles. The Pres. seems to know as much about his muscles as the doctors— probably more!" Franklin's blood pressure after the swim was 260/150—to say the least, alarming. Dr. Bruenn discouraged further forays into the pool.

For several days, Franklin remained idle. "He felt 'executive,'" Daisy wrote, "but didn't want to *do* anything."[5] On December 13, Franklin's previous cardiologist, Dr. Robert Duncan, came to Warm Springs from Bethesda, possibly to administer streptomycin, a potent new antibiotic first used on humans only a month previously at the Mayo Clinic, to treat his multiple bacterial infections.

Ignoring Bruenn's admonitions, Franklin returned to the pool on December 14—balancing the risk of raising his blood pressure with the absolute necessity to regain the ability to stand in his braces. That evening, "[Bruenn and Duncan] seem to be concentrating on the Pres.' heart," Daisy wrote. "He himself said it was a 'cardiac' condition and that his muscles are 'deteriorating,' and that they don't know why."[6]

---

4 *Ibid.*, December 2, 1944.
5 *Ibid.*, December 8, 1944.
6 *Ibid.*, December 15, 1944.

Franklin and Daisy returned to Washington on December 19. "I had quite a talk with Anna about her father's health," Daisy wrote. "It is a very difficult problem & I am entirely convinced that he cannot keep up the present rate—he will kill himself if he tries, and he won't be so very useful to the world then."

By early January, Basil, "Doc," O'Connor, Franklin's friend, former law partner, and the executor of his will, was telling Vice President-elect Harry Truman to "be ready" to assume the presidency, "as the Boss could go at any time."[7] O'Connor canceled a trip to Europe to avoid being overseas when Franklin died.[8]

A cabinet meeting was convened on January 19. "As I sat down beside him I had a sense of his enormous fatigue," Frances Perkins wrote. "He had the pallor, the deep gray color, of a man who had been long ill. He looked like an invalid who has been allowed to see guests for the first time and the guests stayed too long. He supported his head with his hand as though it were too much to hold up. His lips were blue. His hand shook."[9]

Franklin insisted that all thirteen of his grandchildren be in Washington for the inauguration and footed the bill for some of the train tickets. Eleanor said later he seemed to be "realizing full well this would certainly be his last inauguration, perhaps even having a premonition he would not be with us very long."[10] Franklin also insisted his eldest son James, stationed in the Philippines, be present. A special executive order had to be drafted. When James arrived, Franklin performed a rite of passage—removing the family ring from his hand and presenting it to his oldest son.[11]

The inauguration was moved to the White House south portico from its traditional location on the Capitol steps. There were no marching bands, no floats, nor inaugural balls. When asked why, Franklin replied, "Who

---

7 O'Connor confided the conversation to Dr. Hal "Toby" Raper, the son of Warm Springs medical chief Dr. Stuart Raper, in 1964. Personal communication of the author with Dr. Hal "Toby" Raper, July 2018.

8 Hassett, W.D., *Off the Record with F.D.R*, New Brunswick, NJ: Rutgers University Press, 1958, 328.

9 Perkins, 393.

10 Goodwin, 571.

11 The ring has since been passed down another generation and is presently in the possession of James' eldest son (Personal communication between the author and James Roosevelt, Jr.).

is there to parade?"[12] The changes were made to accommodate his failing health. At this point he was far too weak to "walk" to the lectern with Jimmy at his side as he had done at his three previous inaugurals.

"The last time I saw Father I realized something was terribly wrong," James later wrote. "He looked awful and, regardless of what the doctors said I knew in my heart his days were numbered. It was a bitterly cold, raw day, and Father insisted on going to the ceremony without an overcoat. I begged Father to throw his naval cape over his shoulders but he brushed aside my suggestion."[13] As he had done in New York City in November, Franklin used the frigid weather as a stimulant to maintain mental alertness.

Lengthy speech drafts were submitted by Sam Rosenman, Archibald MacLeish, and Robert Sherwood—none of them aware that Franklin was unable to stand anywhere near long enough to deliver remarks of such length. "The President combined them into a speech which was shorter than any of the three drafts," Rosenman later wrote.[14] Eight hundred formal invitations were sent out—five thousand people showed up. One of them was Lucy Mercer Rutherfurd, who stood unobtrusively on the White House lawn. Daisy Suckley later visited her at her sister's home to fill in details of the events at the White House.[15]

Before Franklin started speaking, Secretary of State Edward Stettinius Jr. and Henry Wallace thought they saw him undergoing some sort of seizure, probably from pain.[16] "His whole body shook, especially his right arm, which grasped the rail of the reading stand," Wallace wrote.[17]

"I *think* two men, [Secret Service agents] G. Spaman & C. Fredericks, lifted him out of his chair to an upright position," Daisy Suckley wrote. "He held on to the handles of the desk with both hands. During the first part of the speech

---

12 Goodwin, 672.
13 Roosevelt and Shalett, 354–355.
14 Rosenman, 517. FDR had also shortened his State of the Union speech earlier in the month to deliver it on the radio rather than live, as had been customary (Rosenman, 515).
15 While in Washington, Lucy customarily stayed at her sister Violetta's home at 2238 O Street. Tragically, Violetta put a gun to her head in 1947 after learning of her husband's infidelity.
16 Lelyveld, J., *His Final Battle: The Last Months of Franklin Roosevelt.* New York: Knopf, 2016, 263.
17 *Ibid.*

it looked as though his right arm was straining a good deal, it was trembling. But that all stopped."

Franklin was sworn in by Chief Justice Harlan F. Stone and began speaking at 12:15 p.m. His 559-word address lasted just over five minutes—its somber, prophetic tone reminiscent of Abraham Lincoln's Gettysburg Address.[18] The fourth sentence began "As I stand here," perhaps a self-congratulatory nod to the effort he had had to make just to be able to deliver the speech. Never again did he even attempt to stand in public.

Franklin summed up his struggle over the previous eighteen months.

> "I remember that my old schoolmaster, Dr. Peabody,[19] said, in days that seemed to us then to be secure and untroubled, 'Things in life will not always run smoothly. Sometimes we will be rising toward the heights—then all will seem to reverse itself and start downward.'"

"When the speech was over ... Jimmy asked if he wanted the chair [his wheelchair], his answer was 'Oh, no, I'm very comfortable,'" Daisy Suckley wrote.[20] But Franklin was *not* comfortable. "Just before he proceeded to the reception in the State Dining Room, Father and I were alone for a few minutes in the Green Room," James recalled. "He was thoroughly chilled and the same type of pain, though somewhat less acute, that had bothered him in San Diego was stabbing him again.[21] He gripped my arm and said, 'Jimmy, I can't take this unless you get me a stiff drink.' I said I would and as I started out he called to me, 'You'd better make it straight.' I brought him a tumbler full of whisky, which he drank as if it were medicine. In all my life I never had seen Father take a drink in that manner ... I was deeply disturbed. I ran around like a chicken with my head cut off trying to get to one of his physicians or someone close to him to tell me what was wrong with Pa. The only person who would admit to me that Father was a sick man was George Fox [Franklin's medical aide since 1933] ... Had I discussed the matter that day with Bill Hassett, his devoted secretary, or Basil O'Connor, they would have told me they shared my fears. Regardless of all the soothing talk from the doctors, they felt, as I

---

18 It was the second-shortest inaugural address in American history. Washington's second inaugural in 1796 was a mere 135 words.
19 Peabody died only two months before, on November 17, 1944. He had presided over the religious services at FDR's first three inaugurals, as well as his wedding to Eleanor in 1905.
20 Ward, *Closest Companion*, 388.
21 Far more probably the pain came from Franklin's lower spine, as he had experienced in Bremerton.

did, that Father's days were surely numbered. It showed in the way he talked, the way he looked. There was a drawn, almost ethereal look about him. At times his old zestfulness was there, but often—particularly when he let his guard down—he seemed thousands of miles away." Jimmy was unknowingly describing his father's seizures.

"Did you get a good look at the President?" Edith Wilson commented to Frances Perkins. "Oh, it frightened me. He looks exactly like my husband looked when he went into his decline."[22]

"Of the various things we discussed on that last time I saw Father, one subject alone stirred the old fire in him," James wrote. "That was his prospective trip to Yalta to confer with Stalin and Churchill. Father felt deeply and intensely that the hopes for a decent and just peace depended largely on what he would be able to negotiate with Stalin at Yalta. As he talked about it, one almost could see him throw off his fatigue as he became stimulated with the thought of the challenging task that faced him."[23]

---

22 Goodwin, 573.
23 *Ibid.*, 355–356.

■ Chapter 25
■ The Sick Man at Yalta

Franklin departed for Yalta just thirty-three hours after delivering his inaugural address. Critical issues studded the agenda—partitioning postwar Europe, Poland's status, conditions for Soviet entry into the war against Japan, and the terms for the U.S.S.R. to participate in the United Nations. He came to the summit at a disadvantage. Stalin and Churchill both knew they would be negotiating with a man who would soon be dead.

Franklin would have preferred the conference to be held along the Mediterranean, but Stalin, citing doctors' advice, insisted on a setting closer to Moscow. The three leaders settled on Yalta, a war-ravaged Crimean resort city on the Black Sea. Churchill arrived first and sent word to Franklin: "If we had spent ten years on research, we could not have picked a worse place in the world than Yalta. It is good for typhus and deadly lice, which thrive in these parts."

Franklin's journey took nearly two weeks—the first eight days aboard the cruiser USS *Quincy* to reach Malta in the Mediterranean, then a 1,200-mile flight at low altitude to the Crimean village of Saki, touching down at noon on February 3.[1] The final leg was an eighty-mile, six-hour drive over unpaved roads lined with soldiers to the conference site, Yalta's Livadia Palace.

During briefings en route, Franklin's demeanor unsettled his military advisers, whose ranks included Admiral Ernest J. King, commander in chief of the U.S. fleet. The President listened but did not speak. To King, Franklin seemed to want to get rid of his uniformed advisers, so meetings were often abbreviated.

"I was disturbed by his appearance," Jimmy Byrnes wrote in his memoir. "I feared his illness was not entirely due to a cold and expressed this concern to Mrs. Boettinger [Franklin's daughter Anna]. She thought my opinion arose from observing him during the moving pictures, when she usually sat on one side of the President and I the other."[2] By this time, Anna was well aware of

---

1 Howard Bruenn estimated the altitude to be between 6,000 and 8,000 feet. Another concession to Franklin's fragile cardiac status.
2 Byrnes, J.F., *Speaking Frankly*. Harper & Brothers, 1947, 22.

her father's tenuous medical condition, writing to her husband, John, "My fear is, of course, that [Father] will have a terrific let-down when he gets home, and possibly crack under it as he did last year ... but all we can do is hold our fingers crossed."[3]

"So far as I could see," Byrnes wrote, "the President made little preparation for the Yalta Conference. Not until the day before we landed at Malta did I learn we had on board a very complete file of studies and recommendations prepared by the State Department. I am sure the failure to study them was due to the President's illness. And I am sure that only President Roosevelt, with his intimate knowledge of the problems, could have handled the situation so well with so little preparation."[4]

Franklin's first three nights at Yalta were disrupted by a persistent wracking cough severe enough to rouse him from sleep. Dr. Bruenn prescribed syrup of terpin hydrate and codeine. On February 8, the focus on Poland's fate left the president "greatly fatigued ... His color was poor (gray) but examination showed that his lungs were clear and the heart sounds were of good quality— regular in rhythm and rate (84/min)," Bruenn later wrote. But Franklin had been feasting on salt-laden caviar provided by Stalin in unlimited quantities. The sodium load further challenged his failing heart, causing *pulsus alternans*, a life-threatening condition during which the heart toggles between strong and weak beats. Bruenn was forced to curtail Franklin's schedule. For the remainder of the conference, he saw no visitors before noon and rested for at least an hour before any afternoon session.[5] Previously unknown film shot at Yalta by Colonel Joseph Mayton, translator for General George Marshall[6] shows a coughing, cadaverous figure. Even so, cardiovascular disease was not Franklin's primary medical liability.

Franklin's major limiting factors at Yalta were neurological. Aside from frequent seizures, he was encumbered by metabolic encephalopathy—"brain fog"—due to continuous pain, severe hypertension, multiple organ failure, and the side effects and interactions of the cocktail of drugs being used to treat those ailments.[7] Encephalopathy diminishes the ability to maintain attention

---

3 Anna to John Boettinger, February 14, 1945, Box 6, Anna Halsted papers, FDRL.
4 Byrnes, 23.
5 Bruenn, "Clinical Notes."
6 https://www.youtube.com/watch?v=CYljU7zZQIM.
7 At the very least, digitalis to improve heart function, penicillin and streptomycin for infection, phenobarbital for seizures, and opiates for pain.

and multitask—a significant impairment for a man who prided himself as the hub of the wheel in every important matter of policy.

Churchill's physician, Lord Moran, noted an uncharacteristic tendency of the President to be touchy and irritable if forced to concentrate for very long. Moran was surprised by Franklin's lack of drive and Prime Minister Churchill's seeming inability to make him understand that Stalin was playing them against each other. "Again and again the President seems to have fallen into traps set by Stalin—and to some extent even by Churchill—losing points he would never have conceded had he been in good health and with his earlier ability to control situations," Moran wrote. "Everyone seemed to agree that the President has gone to bits physically. He intervened very little in the discussions, sitting with his mouth open. If he has sometimes been short of the facts about the subject under discussion his shrewdness has covered this up. Now, they say, the shrewdness is gone, and there is nothing left ... To a doctor's eye, the President appears to be a very sick man. He has all the symptoms of hardening of the arteries of the brain in an advanced stage and I give him only a few months to live.[8] Winston is puzzled and distressed. The President no longer seems to the P.M. to take an intelligent interest in the war; often he does not seem to read the papers the P.M. gives him."[9]

"The President, now failing fast, was far too ill to respond to his old friend's admonitions of the folly of allowing the Russians to overrun more of Europe than necessary," Chief of the British Imperial Staff Lord Alanbrooke noted.[10] Writing in *Life* magazine in 1948, William Bullitt, who had been America's first ambassador to the Soviet Union, blamed Franklin's health for a subpar performance. "At Yalta, the Soviet dictator welcomed the weary Franklin Roosevelt, indeed he was more than tired. He was ill," Bullitt wrote. "Little was left of the physical and mental rigor that had been his when he entered the White House in 1933. Frequently he had difficulty in formulating his thoughts, and greater difficulty in expressing them consecutively. But he still held to his determination to appease Stalin."[11] Franklin was sure of one thing—without Stalin, the United Nations could never come to fruition.

8 Moran, *Churchill at War 1940-1945*. London: Basic Books, 2002, 272, 277.
9 Moran, Churchill Taken from the Diaries of Lord Moran: The Struggle for Survival, 1940-1965. London: Constable, 1966, 43.
10 Barach, A., "Franklin Roosevelt's Illness: Effect on History." *New York State Journal of Medicine* 1977;77(13):2156; from Bryant, A., *Triumph in the West*. Doubleday and Co., 1959.
11 Evans, Chapter 5, reference 134.

Diplomat Averell Harriman argued at first that the President carried on the negotiations "with his usual skill and perception,"[12] but later equivocated. "I was terribly shocked at the change from after our talks in Washington after the November elections," Harriman wrote. "The signs of deterioration seemed to me unmistakable ... At Yalta I believe he didn't have the strength to be quite as stubborn as he liked to be. I suppose that if FDR had been in better health, he might have held out longer and got his way on a number of detailed points. But I don't believe it would have made any difference, say, in the Poland question."[13]

Frequent seizures also affected Franklin's performance, which explains why some observers found him lucid and competent while others were struck by a quite different and alarming state of affairs. Along with everyone else, Churchill did not understand the nature of the neurological events he was witnessing. "His captivating smile, his gay and charming manner had not deserted him, but his face had a transparency, an air of purification, and often there was a far-away look in his eyes," Churchill wrote.[14] Naval aide William Rigdon also saw that look. "Some of us noticed, but without concern, that his lower jaw often hung down as we watched the [motion] pictures," Rigdon wrote.[15]

Assessments of Franklin's performance were not all negative. Among his staunchest supporters were eyewitness observers like Secretary of State Edward Stettinius Jr. "I wish to emphasize that at all times from Malta through the Crimean conference and the Alexandria meeting I always found him to be mentally alert and fully capable of dealing with each situation as it developed," Stettinius later wrote.[16]

"Our leader was ill at Yalta, but he was effective," translator Charles "Chip" Bohlen wrote in 1973. "The outcome of the conference was not adversely affected by FDR's health ... I so believed at the time and still so believe."[17] "I do

12 Harriman, A.W., *Military Situation in the Far East*, Harriman Statement, MacArthur Hearings, pt. V, 3330.
13 Harriman, W.A., Abel, A., Special Envoy to Churchill and Stalin, 1941–1946, 388–390. From Barach, 2154–2157.
14 Crispell and Gomez, 125.
15 Evans, Chapter 5, reference 134.
16 Stettinius, E.R. Jr., Roosevelt and the Russians: The Yalta Conference. New York: Doubleday, 1949, 73.
17 Bohlen, C.E., *The Transformation of American Foreign Policy*. New York: Norton, 1969, 172–173.

not know any case where he really gave anything away to the Soviets because of his ill health. He seemed to be guided very heavily by his advisers and took no step independently."[18] Of course, Franklin's most influential Soviet affairs adviser at Yalta was Alger Hiss—later exposed as a Soviet spy.

The most glowing assessment of all, though surely not the most honest, came from Howard Bruenn. "Despite the demands made upon him, his mental clarity was truly remarkable," Bruenn wrote to Ross McIntire in 1946. "His memory for past and recent events was unimpaired and his recollections of detail was such as to continually impress me when compared with some of his associates ten and twenty years younger than himself."[19]

Despite criticism over Soviet dominance over Poland, which by February 1945 had progressed beyond Franklin's ability to reverse,[20] the strongest indictment of Franklin's performance at Yalta arises from two agreements not revealed until weeks after the final communiqué was issued. One was the inclusion of two additional Soviet states, Ukraine and Byelorussia, as voting members of the UN General Assembly. This had little practical effect. The other far more consequential arrangement set the terms by which the Soviets would enter the war against Japan. On the afternoon of February 8, Franklin met privately with Stalin and struck a deal involving China without the knowledge or consent of Nationalist Chinese leader Chiang Kai-shek. In essence, the Soviets would be given all the territory that Czarist Russia had ceded to Japan in the Treaty of Portsmouth that ended the Russo-Japanese War in 1905.[21] The U.S.S.R. did not declare war on Japan until August 8, four months after FDR's death and two days after the atomic bomb had ravaged Hiroshima.

The two Americans with the greatest understanding of the long-term consequences of the China agreement were Ambassador to China Patrick Hurley, a Republican who had been Secretary of War in the Hoover administration, and General Albert C. Wedemeyer, Chiang Kai-shek's chief of staff after

---

18 *Ibid.*, 44; as quoted in Ferrell, 106.
19 Bruenn to McIntire. Goldsmith, 139.
20 The Curzon Line was established as the eastern border of Poland at the Tehran summit in late 1943. By the time of the meeting at Yalta, Stalin had recognized the puppet government at Lublin and Churchill had met with Stalin in October 1944 to barter political control of the Balkans and Greece. Churchill's report to Parliament after returning from the Crimea was equally or more optimistic than Roosevelt's address to Congress on March 1.
21 President Theodore Roosevelt was awarded the Nobel Peace Prize for successfully negotiating the treaty.

General "Vinegar" Joe Stilwell was recalled. Neither Hurley nor Wedemeyer were at Yalta nor had either been consulted beforehand. The agreement was also withheld from General Douglas MacArthur, military commander of the Pacific theater.

Robert Sherwood defended Franklin's decisions at Yalta concerning Poland but admitted, "Only at the end of seven days of long meetings, covering a whole range of tremendous subjects, did he make a concession which, in my belief, he would not have made if he had not been tired out and anxious to end the negotiations relative to Russia's entry into the war with Japan."[22]

Ambassador Hurley went to Washington after getting wind of the China deal. State Department officials told him no such agreement had been made. On March 8, by his own account, Hurley "went to the White House to have a fight about what had been done."

He had not seen Franklin for over six months. "When the President reached up that fine, firm, strong hand of his to shake hands with me, what I found in my hand was a very loose bag of bones," Hurley wrote. "The skin seemed to be pasted down on his cheek-bones, and you know, all the fight I had in me went out."[23]

At first, Franklin denied any such agreement had been made, but after examining documents which included the "Agreement Regarding Japan," Hurley perceived the agreement as "secretly sabotaging, setting aside and canceling every principle and objective for which the United States professed to be fighting World War II." After much persuasion, Franklin directed Hurley to go to London and Moscow to "ameliorate the betrayal of China and return to the traditional American policy in the Far East." Hurley was in Moscow, preparing to meet Stalin, when Franklin died. He later refused to blame his leader for what he regarded as a blunder. "The sickness of death was already upon President Roosevelt when he attended the Yalta Conference," Hurley wrote. "I am certain that he believed he was telling the truth when he said that no secret agreement such as I described had been entered into at Yalta."[24]

---

22 Sherwood, 854.
23 *Time*, July 2, 1951.
24 Lohbeck, D., *Patrick J. Hurley*. Chicago: Henry Regnery, 1956, 138.

General Wedemeyer was a long-standing anti-Communist and an ardent supporter of Chiang Kai-shek.[25] After a stop in Manila to visit MacArthur, Wedemeyer arrived at the White House on March 8, catching Franklin in the midst of a seizure. "His color was ashen, his face drawn and his jaw drooping," the general wrote. "I had difficulty conveying information to him because he seemed in a daze. Several times I repeated the same idea because his mind did not seem to retain or register."[26] During Franklin's intervals of lucidity, Wedemeyer was able to conduct a disjointed discussion about their common interest in opposing France's colonial intentions in Indochina.[27]

A few days later, War Secretary Henry Stimson asked Wedemeyer his impression of Franklin's condition. "I told him I was shocked to find the President in Never-Never Land most of the time that I spent with him, picking nervously at his food and going off on tangents," Wedemeyer wrote in his 1958 memoir. "The Secretary admonished me quietly but firmly not to mention the President's condition to anyone.... This admonishment was reminiscent of the situation that prevailed when President Wilson was so ill and his condition was not revealed to the American people."[28]

---

25 Wedemeyer came upon his anti-Bolshevik stance during his time in Berlin in 1937 when he was the only American to be trained at the German *Kriegsakademie* in Berlin. He became George Marshall's Chief of Staff and was America's primary expert on German military tactics during the war.
26 Wedemeyer, A.C., *Wedemeyer Reports!*. New York: Henry Holt & Company, 1958, 340.
27 *Ibid.*
28 *Ibid.*, 343.

■ Chapter 26
■ "Pardon Me"

The Yalta summit ended on February 11. Franklin was driven to the Black Sea port of Sevastopol, spent the night aboard Appalachian class USS *Catoctin*, then sailed to Egypt for two days of meetings at Great Bitter Lake with the "three kings"—Farouk of Egypt, Haile Selassie of Ethiopia, and Ibn Saud of Saudi Arabia. He then rendezvoused in Alexandria with Churchill and Secretary of State Edward Stettinius, who had just returned from a meeting in Moscow with Foreign Commissar Vyacheslav Molotov. Franklin's final stop before returning home was Algiers, where a meeting with the Provisional President of France, General Charles de Gaulle, had been arranged. Miffed at not being invited to Yalta, De Gaulle declined the invitation at the last minute.[1]

Franklin spent the first days of his return voyage doing little more than sitting on the deck of *Quincy* with Anna, swaddled in blankets. The ship's mood turned somber with the news that, on the heels of a heart attack the week before, Franklin's Chief of Staff, "Pa" Watson, had died on board *Quincy* from a stroke. The amiable Virginian was a year younger than Franklin and, like him, had been dealing with cardiac and prostate problems.[2]

Sam Rosenman had flown from London to Algiers to help Franklin with the speech he was to give upon his return. Rosenman had hoped to complete the job in time to disembark *Catoctin* at Gibraltar but was unable to engage the president's attention until the ship had almost reached American waters.[3] "It was approximately one month since I had seen [Franklin] last," Rosenman recalled. "I was disheartened by his physical appearance, I had never seen him look so tired. He had lost a great deal more weight; he was listless and apparently uninterested in conversation—he was all burnt out."[4]

The speech was a timely chance for Franklin to sell his dream of a world peace organization—a pitch far too crucial to make on radio or edited film, as he

---

1   Moses, J.B., Cross, W., *Presidential Courage*. New York: W.W. Norton, 1980, 209–210.
2   Watson had suffered a heart attack while at Tehran in November, 1943. McIntire files FDRL.
3   Rosenman, 522.
4   *Ibid.*

had done for his State of the Union address less than two months earlier. For the first time, ill health was going to force him to deliver a major address while seated.

Franklin's first public acknowledgment of his disability had to appear to be spontaneous. The master orator and showman who orchestrated every word and gesture of his public appearances would have to commit his opening remarks to memory. It was out of character to say, in effect, "Look at me. I am crippled." He crafted an appeal for empathy, rather than pity, instead. "I hope that you will pardon me for an unusual posture of sitting down during the presentation of what I want to say," he was going to say to a joint session of Congress, "but I know that you will realize that it makes it a lot easier for me in not having to carry about ten pounds of steel around on the bottom of my legs, and also because of the fact that I've just completed a fourteen-thousand-mile trip." Now that the hardest part was over, Franklin summoned Rosenman to begin the tedious business of speechwriting.

Three drafts of the speech were created aboard *Quincy*. Once back in Washington, Franklin and Rosenman were joined by Franklin's son-in-law, John Boettinger, for two more rewrites. The reading copy underwent so many revisions Grace Tully retyped it as a sixth draft.[5] Finally, thirty-one double-spaced pages were placed in a three-ring binder to be carried into the House of Representatives.

Franklin's previous speeches to Congress had usually been given in the evening. But now his mental acuity waned as the day wore on. "Roosevelt was an animated human being from 9:00 a.m. until 1:00 p.m.," biographer Jim Bishop wrote. "Each day, at lunchtime, he appeared to shatter into helpless fragments. The good nature seemed intact, but the body and mind faded in function toward a smiling helplessness."[6] Franklin would give this speech in the early afternoon.

For prior addresses to Congress, Franklin had been stationed at the speaker's podium with his wheelchair out of sight before the audience was permitted into the chamber. This time, the galleries and the floor of the House were filled before he arrived. Speaker pro tempore John McCormick of Massachusetts gave the customary introduction: "Senators and Representatives, I have the great pleasure, the high privilege and the distinguished honor of presenting

---

5 *Ibid.*, 527.
6 Bishop, London Hart-Davis MacGibbon, 1975, 532.

to you the President of the United States." Silence fell as he was wheeled in—a sight most of those present had never witnessed. Franklin was assisted into a comfortable red chair positioned in the area in front of the speaker's rostrum known as the well.

After thunderous applause faded, Franklin began to speak, needing to pause for a second breath to complete his rehearsed opening. Illness had robbed his stentorian voice of its familiar booming resonance. The studiedly casual opening seemed to put the audience at ease—but as he looked down to read his remarks in the binder, he began having difficulty finding words on the pages before him. In the past, he compensated for his visual deficiencies by using his right hand as a stylus to keep his place for speeches excerpted on film or broadcast over the radio. Now, before a live audience, he was unable to read and speak at the speed needed to deliver a fluent, coherent address.[7]

Only the guile and experience of a master orator who had delivered thousands of public addresses prevented complete disaster. Every sentence became a potential grammatical nightmare that required adjustment on the fly. He often improvised at length to give himself mental rest and find his place. Halfway through, he muttered about wishing to be done in an hour—a torturous time that must have seemed an eternity. Some of the rambling improvisations made no sense. During others he committed political faux pas—referring to Charles de Gaulle as a "prima donna" and to Saudi Arabian King Ibn Saud's intransigence regarding ethnic problems in the Middle East.

After the speech, reporters made a beeline for Vice President Harry Truman. It had become abundantly clear Truman would be assuming the presidency a lot sooner than had been anticipated. When asked his opinion of the address, the blunt Missourian sarcastically quipped, "One of the greatest ever given."[8]

"I was dismayed at the halting, ineffective manner of delivery," Sam Rosenman wrote. "He ad-libbed a great deal—as frequently as I had ever heard him. Some of his extemporaneous remarks were wholly irrelevant, and some of them almost bordered on the ridiculous.... It was quite obvious that the great fighting eloquence and oratory that distinguished him in his campaign only four months before were lacking."[9] Rosenman was "lower than I have ever seen

---

7 In 1944, Franklin did not give his State of the Union speech live to Congress due to the "flu." This time he was unable because he couldn't stand long enough to deliver the speech.

8 Drury, A., *A Senate Journal 1943-1945*. New York: McGraw Hill, 1963, 373.

9 Rosenman, 527.

him," Jonathan Daniels wrote. "He had a feeling that the President's ad-libbing had made a mess of the speech and that some of the things he had put in were going to have a very bad reaction."[10]

"This speech was the first indication to many that something may be gravely wrong with the President," journalist John Gunther wrote. "He ad-libbed a great deal. In fact, never in his whole career had he ever ad-libbed so much in an important speech; he departed from his prepared text no fewer than forty-nine times. This phenomenon was too disconcerting to those who were worried about his condition."[11]

Word-by-word comparison of the reading copy with the audio recording revealed a pattern which showed how the stumbles, repetitions, and substitutions were due to omissions of smaller words and an inability to see the left side of larger ones.[12] Ad-libs usually occurred when Franklin lost his place and missed the left margin, or after he turned a page.[13] The holes in Franklin's left-side vision were most likely due to the metastatic melanoma invading the right side of his brain.

The White House went into damage control mode, though most reports in the press and by the major news services were surprisingly favorable. "Congressmen generally thought he looked thin, but his voice was resilient and he had a tan from the sea voyage," the New York *Daily News* reported. One exception was the anti-Roosevelt *Chicago Tribune*. "The usual smile and waves of the hand were absent as members roundly applauded his entrance.... The lengthy speech was delivered in a mechanical tone of voice which seldom was raised until the final paragraph. Delivery was sometimes marked by hesitancy as the President obviously lost his place several times," said the paper. "Despite the wide variations from the text, nothing will appear in the

---

10 Daniels, 267.

11 Gunther, 363–364.

12 www.fdrsdeadlysecret.blogspot.com has links to the audio recording and an annotated recording of the speech that shows all the errors. A fabulous neurological detective story.

13 A fascinating incident recorded by Daisy Suckley in her diary on January 14, 1945 inadvertently also documented Franklin's visual loss. A classic neurological examination technique for left-sided visual loss is to ask a patient to read the word "northwestern." Impaired patients will see it as "western" or "stern." In this case Daisy noted: "FDR called up at 5 minutes of two—He had mistaken the time on his clock & had just come down for his lunch" (Ward, *Closest Companion*, 381). Visual loss had caused him to not see the first digit in "11," thus at 1:55 Franklin believed the time to be 11: 55.

Congressional Record except the President's prepared speech, unless the White House says otherwise."

Press Secretary Jonathan Daniels struggled to transcribe the speech for official release. Robert Sherwood later commented how daunting it had been to try to make sense of portions of a major address *after* it had been given. The audio recording was emended to remove some of the stumbles, repetitions, and coughing. Films of the event were more drastically edited. Two movie cameras positioned to Franklin's right had been rolling, one at close range and the other in the gallery. Only a few minutes of footage was deemed acceptable for newsreels. The remainder wound up on the cutting room floor.[14] The March 1, 1945, address is one of the most important of Franklin's speeches for which no complete visual record exists.

By March 1945, the fourth estate was accustomed to a failing president's lapses. At a press conference, Bert Andrews of the New York *Herald Tribune* asked Franklin to comment on remarks about the United Nations by former Minnesota governor Harold Stassen, whom he had appointed a delegate to that body's opening session, scheduled for April 25 in San Francisco.

"Stassen?" Franklin asked. "Who's Stassen?"

A hurried "Thank you, Mr. President!" ended the conference. None of this appeared in the official transcript. As reporters were filing out, May Craig of the Portland, Maine, *Press Herald* turned to a group of her colleagues, including Walter Trohan, and asked "What do you make of him?" "He's like the last leaf on the tree," Burt Hulen of *The New York Times* answered. In another instance, "Franklin baffled assembled reporters by going into a long exposition on flood control, which certainly had no relation to the war and little to the public interest. Again, the conference was cut short."[15] Trohan waited until 1975 to include all of this in his memoir.

Walter Trohan toed a fine line between reporting the truth about Franklin's health and being banished from the White House press corps. Over the years, he had developed a cordial relationship with Franklin, who was well aware of the conservative politics of his newspaper and its owner/publisher, "Colonel"

---

14 At this writing, an unedited video of the speech has not been located. It is unlikely that it will ever be.

15 Trohan, *Political Animals*, 190.

Robert R. "Bertie" McCormick, an alumnus of Groton School and Yale.[16] Trohan publicized his scoops by leaking them to the FBI and other journalists.[17] His papers are housed at the Herbert Hoover Library in North Branch, Iowa, uncensored, unlike those in Hyde Park where Daisy Suckley reigned supreme. His 1975 memoir, *Political Animals*, has some factual errors and misspellings (i.e., "Sterling") but still abounds with unique tidbits and anecdotes. Among the most tantalizing is his exposure of Franklin's urologist who would treat his prostate cancer, William Calhoun Stirling.

---

16 Trohan papers, Herbert Hoover Library, North Branch, IA.
17 Trohan gave his inside information about Lucy Mercer to journalist Westbrook Pegler, who broke the story in a series of press releases. Pegler's story went nowhere, probably out of respect for Eleanor. Even the *Chicago Tribune* refused to print stories about Franklin's love life. Colonel McCormick was quoted as saying "We don't do business that way."

■ Chapter 27
■ The End

Franklin was the honored guest at the annual White House Correspondents Association Dinner on March 22, 1945, at the Statler Hotel in Washington. Comedians Danny Kaye, Fanny Brice, and Jimmy Durante provided the entertainment. Decades later, UPI correspondent Allen Drury told Franklin's biographer Jim Bishop he was saddened by watching Franklin being wheeled into the packed banquet hall. "He looked old, thin, scrawny-necked, and he stared at the tables with a vacant expression," Drury said. "He didn't even respond to the ruffles and flourishes of the band and the deafening applause…. When laughter engulfed the room, the Boss cupped his ear and asked a table companion to repeat the joke. A moment later he would stare out at nothing: the vague expression in his eyes, his mouth hanging open. At the close of the entertainment, he was expected to say something. Microphones were placed before him. It was embarrassing. 'I will say something. I will speak about humanity,' Franklin muttered. 'We all love humanity. You love humanity. I love humanity. In the name of humanity, I will give you a headline story. I am calling off tomorrow's press conference.'"[1]

Franklin went to Hyde Park on Saturday, March 24. The next morning—Palm Sunday—he and Eleanor, with Fala in tow, drove to Rhinebeck for a visit to Daisy Suckley to see her new litter of puppies. "The President looks terribly badly," Daisy wrote. "So tired that every word seems to be an effort. They stayed for about 3/4 of an hour, Mrs. R. doing her best to get him started home to see some people at six—more people for dinner—He just can't stand this strain indefinitely. Thank heavens he gets off to [Warm Springs] on Thursday night after another long day in Washington."[2]

Walter Trohan was at press headquarters at the Palmer House Hotel in Poughkeepsie early Palm Sunday afternoon when calls began to swamp the local telephone exchange. He took a taxi to Springwood to investigate but the Secret Service turned him around. The next day, he learned "on the best authority"—possibly Secret Service agent Mike Reilly—that the president had had a stroke or cerebral hemorrhage. Trohan's source said Franklin was

---

1 Bishop, 519–520.
2 *Suckley Diary*, March 25, 1945.

unconscious for some time, causing physicians to fear the event had been fatal. But he revived, and within hours, seemed back to normal. No cerebral hemorrhage could possibly have been so transient. The event was a grand mal seizure. Years later, White House butler Alonzo Fields wrote of "rumors that the President had had an attack at Hyde Park during his stay there during Holy Week."[3]

Franklin's calendar and Daisy Suckley's diary are blank for three days after the Palm Sunday seizure. On Wednesday, March 28, an attendant wheeled Franklin into his library.[4] White House aide George Elsey, whom Franklin knew well, was at work selecting books to take to Warm Springs. When Elsey rose to greet him, Franklin gave no indication of recognition, looked around, and told his attendant to wheel him out.[5]

Grace Tully witnessed the aftermath of another seizure on March 29 during Franklin's brief stop in Washington on the way to Warm Springs. "We had been waiting for the Boss in the oval study and when he was wheeled in I was so startled I almost burst into tears," Tully wrote. "In two hours he seemed to have failed dangerously. His face was ashen, highlighted by the darkening shadows under the eyes and with his cheeks drawn gauntly."[6]

Another dramatic report of a visual problem at this time came from Jonathan Daniels. "In one of my books I told about the last time I saw Roosevelt when Archie MacLeish and I had to go up and see him about that business of those two extra votes for the Russian states," Daniels recalled. "MacLeish and I worked out the statement together and we had to go to see the President just before he went off to Warm Springs. And the tragic thing was (and the toughest moment of my life), Roosevelt made a change up here—we were all of us very concerned about him at that moment—and we got off the elevator and we realized that the change he'd made up here, made it essential that a change be made down here; but it was a matter of such importance that despite his distressing condition, we felt we had to go back and say, 'Mr. President, look.' And that was a damn tough walk back."[7]

---

3 Fields, A., *My 21 Years in the White House*. New York and Greenwich, CT: Fawcett Crest, 1961, 21.
4 Daisy Suckley noted his last visit to the FDRL was between 3:00 and 4:30. Ward, *Closest Companion*, 401.
5 Evans, 109.
6 Tully, 357.
7 Oral history of Jonathan Daniels, Harry S. Truman Library.

Franklin was hell-bent on making a 2,800-mile trip to San Francisco to attend the opening meeting of the United Nations on April 25. He expected to address the assemblage from his wheelchair for less than an hour, then, at a local post office, purchase the first example of the postage stamp he had designed for the occasion and to return home.[8] As he had done in December to prepare for his inauguration, Franklin planned a restorative stay in Warm Springs before his trip west.

As Franklin descended the elevator of *Ferdinand Magellan* on March 30, to begin his forty-first visit to the little town he had made famous, locals who had gathered to greet him were stunned at the sight of his physical deterioration. This time there would be no jaunty repartee. Secret Service agent Mike Reilly found him uncharacteristically "heavy," unable to assist as he transferred the emaciated six-foot-three-inch frame, now weighing 145 pounds, into an open car for the customary parade past Georgia Hall to the Little White House. Railroad agent Charles "C.J." Pless later commented that Franklin was "the worst-looking man I ever saw that was still alive. Just like a setting up dead man"[9]

On March 31, Daisy Suckley and Howard Bruenn sat down for a heart-to-heart talk: "Miss Suckley, you realize that like all people who work with the man—I love him," Bruenn said. "If he told me to jump out of the window, I would do it, without hesitation."[10]

"He, or Doctor McIntire, or *someone*, should put it very plainly to F.D.R. him-self." Daisy responded. "F.D.R.'s one really great wish is to get this international organization for peace started. Nothing else counts next to that. That is the means by which they must make him take care of himself, 'You want to carry out the United Nations plan? Without your health, you will not be able to do it. Therefore—take care of yourself.'"[11]

"He must reduce his hours of work & not break the new schedule," Daisy wrote. "He should take 2-3 months off to get well, but if he can't do that, he can and must fit his workday to his strength—if he is to live through these trying days. It has come to that point, and I think the doctors believe it

---

8 Hassett, 330.
9 Asbell, B., *When FDR Died*. New York: Holt Rinehart and Winston, 1961, 23.
10 Each would protect Franklin's health secrets for nearly half a century after his death. Daisy died in 1992 at age 98, Bruenn in 1994, at 90.
11 *Suckley Diary*, March 31, 1945.

though they have not said it to me.... We had lunch at one, & he ate well.... After a while he went off to his room for an hour before dinner. He looks depressed, both physically & mentally, and it hurts one not to be able to do much for him but to be ready & waiting if anything turns up."[12]

Franklin attended Easter services on April 1. His encephalopathy was such that he could hold neither a prayer book nor his glasses for more than a few minutes without dropping them.[13] He later told Daisy he had not been able to hear a word of the service, likely due to deafness from streptomycin, a yet-to-be reported side effect of the newly discovered antibiotic his team of doctors had prescribed for him.[14,15]

Franklin's spinster cousins devised a pathetic ritual to force-feed him. "I get the gruel & Polly & I take it to him," Daisy wrote on April 4. "I sit on the edge of the bed & he 'puts on an act': he is too weak to raise his head, his hands are weak, he must be fed! So I proceed to feed him with a tea spoon & he loves it! Just to be able to turn from his world problems & behave like a complete nut for a few moments, with an appreciative audience laughing with him & at him, both!

When he can't smile & joke, he is really pretty sick—we are so happy over his improvement in less than a week. Polly confessed that when she saw him last Thursday, she didn't think he would live to go to the San Francisco Conference. She feels entirely differently now, for she sees he can still 'come back' in a remarkable manner."

Gruel is nothing more than oatmeal cooked for five hours.[16] Bruenn had instructed the spinster cousins to feed it to Franklin throughout the day to supplement his caloric intake. It did little but dam up in his blocked intestines.

On the morning of April 9, Franklin's spirits rose. Lucy Rutherfurd was coming to visit him from her estate in Aiken, South Carolina, bringing portraitist

---

12 *Ibid.*
13 This refers to a phenomenon known to neurologists in patients with severe encephalopathy known as motor impersistence.
14 Lomazow, S., "Was Franklin Delano Roosevelt (1882–1945) Treated with Streptomycin?" *Journal of Medical Biography* February 2010;18(1):61.
15 Ross McIntire admitted to Roosevelt's difficulty with hearing in his 1951 interview with *U.S. News and World Report.*
16 Daisy Bonner interview with Margaret and Bert Price, *Atlanta Journal,* April 12, 1950. Westbrook Pegler papers, box 68, Herbert Hoover Library.

Elizabeth Shoumatoff so Franklin could sit for her. The artist had painted him in 1943.[17] Franklin, Daisy, Fala, and a Secret Service agent/driver went to Macon, where he expected to meet Lucy and her companions—Shoumatoff had invited a photographer, Nicholas Robbins, along. They missed connections, and the president spent the better part of the day searching for his love.

Lucy was expecting to be met. "Nobody loves us, nobody cares for us," she told Shoumatoff and Robbins in mock disappointment.[18] The wayward wanderers crossed paths five miles north of Warm Springs outside of a general store where the Aiken party arrived to find Franklin and Daisy drinking Coca-Cola, surrounded by a crowd of onlookers.

On the evening of April 11, Treasury Secretary Henry Morgenthau stopped at Warm Springs on his way back from Florida after visiting his ailing wife. Morgenthau observed how the president confused names, repeated stories, and had difficulty performing his favorite social ritual of mixing drinks. "His hands shook so that he started to knock the glasses over, and I had to hold each as he poured the cocktail.... I noticed that he took the two cocktails and then seemed to feel a little better."[19,20]

White House public relations director David Noyes had observed the same phenomenon on March 20, 1945. "[Franklin] put a cigarette in his holder to light it in the usual way," Noyes wrote. "Unable to connect the match, his hand shaking badly, he opened the desk drawer, placed his bent elbow inside, partly closed the drawer, and got a firm hold on his hand."[21]

On April 12, Franklin awoke with a mild headache and a stiff neck. The first sign of the disaster that would soon follow. His mornings were still blessed with enough physical strength and mental clarity to enable him to sign stacks of official documents in a barely readable hand. Bill Hassett had developed a ritual he jokingly named "doing the laundry," setting freshly signed documents

17 The portrait was intended as a gift for Lucy's daughter Barbara, whom Roosevelt referred to as his godchild. Barbara bore an unmistakable resemblance to her father, Winthrop Rutherfurd, removing any idea Franklin was her real father.

18 Shoumatoff, E., *FDR's Unfinished Portrait.* University of Pittsburgh Press, Pittsburgh, PA: 1990, 101.

19 *Morganthau Diary*, April 11, 1945, FDRL.

20 FDR's tremor came from a combination of problems. There was probably a hereditary component (Anna had it in later life), exacerbated by an encephalopathy from a multitude of medical problems.

21 Ferrell, 111.

throughout the Little White House for the ink to dry.[22] Franklin signed a bill into law and dictated a few letters to Grace Tully in response to reports that Stalin was reneging on commitments made at Yalta. Ever the avid philatelist, he gave final approval for the stamp he had personally designed to commemorate the opening of the United Nations.[23]

April 12 was a clear, beautiful day in Warm Springs—"Roosevelt weather," as locals had come to call it. The landscape was punctuated by flowering dogwoods, blazing azalea, and pale purple wisteria. Aromas of magnolia and pine and the familiar songs of Carolina wrens and mockingbirds filled the air. Dragonflies flitted about. A mile and a half from the main gate, at the end of a winding forest road, sat two unpretentious guest houses and the modest clapboard Little White House, with its portico and rose-spangled columns. The security "bump gate" and guardhouses manned by armed Marines and Secret Service agents testified to its occupant's importance. The house was high on Pine Mountain to afford a magnificent view from the fantail-shaped rear deck but, owing to its owner's fear of fire, not at the peak, where it would have been beyond the range of hoses.

The rustic three-bedroom structure was decorated with simply designed, finely-constructed furniture made by Val-Kill Industries of Hyde Park, New York, as well as ship models, paintings, and prints amassed by a dedicated and astute collector of naval memorabilia.[24] A small square card table where the president had been working and posing was set for lunch. Cook Daisy Bonner's cheese soufflé was rising in the oven.[25] Frail and ashen, the most powerful man on earth sat, surrounded by the people with whom he was most at ease—his devoted staff, his spinster cousins "Daisy" Suckley and Laura "Polly" Franklin Delano, and, most of all, the romantic love of his life—and vice versa—Lucy Page Mercer Rutherfurd.

Daisy Suckley provided the best account of what happened next.

---

22 Hassett would not use a blotter on presidential documents. His ritual of laying them out to air dry became known as "doing the laundry."

23 After his death on the 12th, the postmaster general successfully raced to redesign the stamp to include Roosevelt's name as a memorial on the 25th.

24 Val-Kill Industries was founded by Eleanor and her friends Nancy Cook, Marion Dickerman and Caroline O'Day in 1927.

25 Bonner interview, *Atlanta Journal*, April 12, 1950, 16.

"[At 1:10 p.m. central war time] F. seemed to be looking for something, his head forward, his hands trembling—I went forward & looked into his face. 'Have you dropped your cigarette?'

"He looked at me with his forehead furrowed in pain and tried to smile. He put his left hand up to the back of his head & said 'I have a terrific pain in the back of my head.'

"He said it distinctly, but so low that I don't think anyone else heard it—My head was not a foot from his—I told him to [put] his head back on his chair—Polly came through the door at that moment. We tilted his chair back, as he was slumping forward, & with Polly and Lucy holding the chair, I took up the telephone & said to the operator ... 'Please get in touch with Dr. Bruenn & ask him to come at once to the President's cottage' and put down the receiver."

Madame Shoumatoff had yelled, "Lucy, Lucy, something has happened!" loudly enough to bring valet Arthur Prettyman from the bedroom and house-boy Irineo "Filipino Joe" Esperancilla from the kitchen.

"They picked up F. but found him a dead weight—not at all the way he usually put his arms around the men's shoulders & carried his own weight on them," Daisy continued. "Polly took F's feet & somehow, between us all, we carried him in to his bed and laid him on three pillows." Polly thought she heard him say "Be careful" as Franklin's military cape dragged across the polished floor.

"I opened his collar & tie & held up the left side of his pillow, rather than move him to the middle of it," Daisy wrote. "I held his right hand. Polly was on his left, her hand on his heart, fanning him." Lucy Rutherfurd put camphor to his nose. "Two or three times he rolled his head from side to side, opened his eyes. Polly thinks he looked at us all in turn. He may have, I could see no signs of real recognition in those eyes—twice he drew up the left side of his face, as if in pain—But this was only a question of 3 or 4 minutes, for he became uncon-scious as far as one could see—His breathing was rather heavy but his heart seemed to be steady & strong, though quick."

Daisy Suckley had implored Madame Shoumatoff to "ask the Secret Service man to call a doctor immediately."[26] The artist found agent-in-charge Jim Beary at his post just outside the doorway. When Beary grasped the grav-ity of the situation, he radioed Secret Service headquarters at nearby Carver

---

26 Asbell, *When FDR Died*, 38.

Cottage. Agent Guy Spaman answered and sprinted to his car to fetch chief agent Mike Reilly and Howard Bruenn at the pool.

A few minutes later, after coming back from the pool for lunch, traveling White House telephone operator Louise "Hacky" Hackmeister checked the switchboard in her cottage on the grounds of the foundation. The Warm Springs operator informed her that the Little White House had called for a doctor. Hacky called back to ask if Dr. Bruenn was wanted for lunch. "I guess I'm not supposed to tell—things are kinda secret," cook Daisy Bonner said. "But it's for the President."[27] Hacky called the poolside phone and alerted Bruenn, who told her to find George Fox and tell him to bring his medical bag. Bruenn was dressed and waiting by the time agent Spaman pulled up for a one-and-a-half mile race up the hill to the Little White House.

At 1:25 p.m., fifteen minutes after the president was stricken, Howard Bruenn ran into the Little White House yelling, to no one in particular, "Get me Admiral McIntire and hold him on the line!"[28] Daisy Suckley was asking the operator to reach the White House to get McIntire when Fox arrived with Bruenn's medical bag in hand. Bruenn found his patient unresponsive, in a deep coma. As Prettyman was getting Franklin out of his clothes, the president stopped breathing—his tongue was blocking his airway. The problem was relieved by anchoring it to the bottom of his mouth with a strip of gauze. As Bruenn examined Franklin and took his blood pressure—greater than 300 over 190—[29] he immediately recognized this event was not transient but rather the irrevocable final chapter in his two-year odyssey, something he and Ross McIntire had known was coming but hadn't expected to happen quite so dramatically.

Franklin's right pupil suddenly dilated, an ominous sign of a hemorrhage expanding in his brain. After about ten minutes of administering medications

---

27 Bonner interview, *Atlanta Journal*, April 12, 1950, 16.

28 Bruenn told PBS in an interview that eventually aired in a 1994 "American Experience" video documentary that he arrived with Roosevelt still seated in his chair and personally carried him to the bedroom. This is contradicted by every other eyewitness report and is simply untrue. Just why he chose to say it is unclear.

29 The alarming blood pressure has often been cited as the cause of Roosevelt's hemorrhage, but, in fact, it was *caused* by it. 300 is the upper limit a blood pressure cuff can measure. The phenomenon of increased blood pressure after severe intracranial hemorrhage was first described by iconic neurosurgeon Harvey Cushing and eponymously bears his name. Cushing's daughter, Betsey, was married to FDR's eldest son, James, between 1930 and 1940 and is acknowledged to have been FDR's favorite daughter-in-law.

to dilate blood vessels and lower blood pressure, Bruenn had a moment to report to McIntire, standing by in Washington.

"He was quite well when I left him this morning," Bruenn told McIntire. "He complained of a slight pain in the neck but now something very acute and severe has happened, sir. It looks to me like a massive brain hemorrhage. At this moment he's stable but there's very little else we can do. I'm afraid we're in for a long siege."[30]

McIntire had had ten minutes to think about what to do next. Despite a fully equipped operating room nearby on the grounds of the foundation and secure medical facilities at Fort Benning in nearby Columbus, he elected to let Franklin spend his last moments in the Little White House. As his patient lay dying, McIntire might have felt relief at avoiding the problem his mentor Cary Grayson had confronted with Woodrow Wilson. Franklin's accelerated decline had brought about the very real prospect of history repeating itself.

Lucy declared, "We must pack and go, the family is arriving by plane and the rooms must be vacant. We must get to Aiken before dark,"[31] heading off to the guest house with Shoumatoff to pack, where they were met by maid Lizzie McDuffie. Photographer Nicholas Robbins was at the Warm Springs Hotel.[32] Shoumatoff phoned him to tell of their imminent departure and that a Secret Service agent would be coming to pick him up.

Within half an hour, Daisy Suckley went to the guest house to see Shoumatoff and Lucy off, just as Spaman pulled up with Robbins. By 2:30 the trio were on the road with Shoumatoff at the wheel of her white Cadillac. Aiken was five hours away.

McIntire phoned Atlanta internist James Paullin, then president of the American Medical Association, telling him to find a neurosurgeon and send him to Warm Springs. Paullin enlisted his colleague Homer Swanson, who got in his car, and headed for Warm Springs.

---

30 FDR underwent a series of events all too familiar to neurologists, known as trans-tentorial herniation, in this case consistent with a rapidly expanding mass in the posterior portion of the right side of the brain.

31 Shoumatoff, 119.

32 Robbins was born Nicholas Katsubinsky. As with so many others, upon his immigration his name was shortened and Americanized. As also happened frequently, the name he chose, "Kobbins," was incorrectly transcribed on the official document as "Robbins."

As McIntire was leaving the White House medical office, he encountered an anxious Anna Boettinger coming off the elevator, hurrying to Bethesda Naval Hospital, where her son Johnny was about to undergo an infusion of penicillin to treat a severe upper respiratory infection, a potentially dangerous procedure in 1945.

"What is it?" Anna asked impatiently.

"Your father has had some sort of seizure," McIntire replied. "He's unconscious. Howard Bruenn has been calling from Warm Springs. Whatever it is, we don't think it will affect his brain."

Just then, Bruenn phoned and Anna asked to speak with him. "This thing," she said. "Will it mean any further paralysis for my father?"

"If that were so, it would not be paralysis which would affect his brain,"[33] he told Anna. Satisfied for the moment, she rushed off to Bethesda.

Eleanor was in her White House study with Charles Taussig, an adviser to the upcoming United Nations conference in San Francisco,[34] when the phone rang. Polly Delano was calling from Warm Springs to tell her that Franklin had had a fainting spell.

Eleanor was used to bad medical news about her husband, so while she surely felt concern, there was no reason to believe this event was any more serious than others. The phone rang again. This time it was Ross McIntire. "He had some sort of spell and passed out. Howard Bruenn is with him," he told her.[35]

Eleanor asked if she should cancel her afternoon plans and come to Georgia. With the press still in the dark, McIntire didn't want to sound a premature alarm and told Eleanor to go about her business.

Wearing an attractive red suit, the First Lady set out for the 17th annual Tea and Entertainment of the Thrift Shops, one of Washington's most fashionable charity events, arriving at four o'clock Washington time (one hour later than Warm Springs), at the Sulgrave Club on Dupont Circle.

---

33 Bishop, 585.
34 That morning, Eleanor announced she would be accompanying her husband to the conference. Asbell, *Mother and Daughter*, 185.
35 Asbell, *When FDR Died*, 50.

Seated at the head table between the organization's chairwoman, Mrs. John Dougherty, and Edith Wilson, Eleanor gave a brief speech, then settled in for a program featuring pianist Evelyn Tyner.

In Warm Springs, Bruenn could do little more than supervise his patient's demise. After an hour or so he was able to break away to update McIntire and smoke a cigarette on the back patio, where he came upon a distraught William Hassett. Bruenn reiterated his concern about "a long siege," probably recalling his recent death watch with "Pa" Watson aboard USS *Quincy*.

By 3:30 p.m. Georgia time, only the most primitive regions of Franklin's brain, those that controlled his breathing, were still functioning. For more than two hours his loud and labored death rattle had at once been torture and reassurance to those hearing it in the living room. Bruenn had again stepped away to phone McIntire when Fox yelled, "Doc Bruenn, Doc Bruenn, get in here right away!" Bruenn handed the phone to Polly and sprinted to the bedside. Franklin's respirations had ceased. Bruenn administered an injection while Fox began artificial respiration. Just then, the front door flew open and Dr. Paullin stormed in after a frantic seventy-mile trip from Atlanta, speeding down back roads in an hour and thirty-five minutes. Paullin reached into his medical bag, drew up a vial of adrenaline into a long-needled glass syringe, located the space between Franklin's left fourth and fifth ribs, and injected the stimulant directly into his heart. After a few heartbeats, the doctors found no pulse or blood pressure, there were no respirations. Bruenn called a halt. In a soft but emphatic tone he declared, "This man is dead!" It was 3:35 p.m. Central War Time (4:35 Washington time). Fala crashed through the screen door at the front of the Little White House and howled.

◼ Chapter 28
◼ Going Home

Ross McIntire's top priority was to expunge any evidence that might expose his twelve-year medical cover-up. He immediately began taking measures to prevent an autopsy, instructing Bruenn to contact a funeral director and select a coffin but to do nothing more until he arrived in Warm Springs.

Bill Hassett tracked down Steve Early at the home of Pa Watson's widow. The men decided to announce the death simultaneously. Pool reporters assigned to cover Franklin in Warm Springs were at a barbeque and minstrel show he was scheduled to attend.[1,2] Bill Hassett summoned the trio to press headquarters at Carver Cottage.[3] "Gentlemen, it is my sad duty to inform you that the President of the United States is dead," he said quietly. "He died at 3:35 o'clock this afternoon, Central Standard Time." Bruenn arrived a few minutes later to "round out the story."[4] The doctor attributed the president's death to "a massive cerebral hemorrhage," likening the event to a bolt of lightning. "One minute he was there and laughing, the next minute—wham!" Bruenn told the stunned reporters.

"Did you see this coming?" one of them asked.

"This wasn't the sort of thing you could forecast," Bruenn replied. "Doctors can't just say, 'This man is going to have a cerebral [hemorrhage].' It didn't happen that way. He'd been feeling fine. He was awfully tired when we first came down here. You saw him the other day—wasn't he in fine spirits?" Merriman Smith of the United Press answered that question years later. "Yes, the president was in fine spirits that day, but he looked unhealthy."[5]

---

1 Harold Oliver of the Associated Press, Merriman Smith of the United Press, and Robert Nixon of the International News Service.
2 The reporters, who came to be known as the "Three Musketeers," were awaiting Franklin's appearance at a barbeque and minstrel show that had been organized by Franklin's old friend, Ruth Stevens. They had thought they were being summoned for an announcement of the end of the war in Europe.
3 The press headquarters was located at Carver Cottage on the grounds of the foundation.
4 Asbell, *When FDR Died*, 73.
5 Smith, M., 183–184.

In Washington, Early called the Sulgrave Club and asked to speak with Mrs. Roosevelt, telling her only to return to the White House as soon as possible. Eleanor had already intuited the purpose of the call. "In my heart I knew what had happened, but one does not actually formulate these terrible thoughts until they are spoken," she later wrote.[6]

The First Lady returned to the dais, waited for a pause in the performance, and excused herself to a standing ovation. At the White House she found Early holding back tears. "I'm so sorry to have to inform you that the president slipped away at 4:35," Early told Eleanor. "Dr. Bruenn was with him but there was nothing he could do."[7]

Protocol dictated that the secretary of state must inform the vice president but Steve Early took it upon himself to have Eleanor break the news. Harry Truman was on Capitol Hill on his way to the "board of education," Speaker Sam Rayburn's regular bourbon-and-branch-water-laced afternoon political soiree. Early left a message at Rayburn's office for Truman to call him as soon as he arrived. When Truman did so, the press secretary calmly told him he was needed at the White House. Thinking he had been tapped for a special assignment, Truman excused himself and told Rayburn he would return shortly. Evading his Secret Service agent, the unknowing thirty-third president briskly walked out to Independence Avenue SE and hailed his government limousine for the mile and a half ride to the White House.

The grief-stricken faces of the White House staff and Roosevelt family members in Eleanor's second-floor study gave Truman the first hint of what he was about to learn—news he'd been dreading since taking office. Eleanor laid her hand on Truman's shoulder. "Harry," she said. "The president is dead!"

"For a moment, I could not bring myself to speak," Truman recalled. "The last news we had had from Warm Springs was [that the president was] apparently doing so well that no member of his family, and not even his personal physician, was with him. All this flashed through my mind before I found my voice."[8]

"Is there anything I can do for you?" Truman asked.

---

6 Roosevelt, E., *This I Remember*. New York: Harper and Brothers, 1949, 344.
7 During Steve Early's press conference, "slipped away" was misheard as "slept away" by a number of reporters and their papers wrote that FDR had died in his sleep.
8 Truman, H., *Memoirs, Vol. I, Year of Decisions*. Garden City: Doubleday, 1955, 412.

"No, sir, is there anything I can do for you?" Eleanor replied. "You're the one who's in trouble now!"

A bawling Secretary of State, Edward Stettinius, appeared. Truman instructed him to convene the cabinet—then approved the use of a military plane to fly the First Lady, Steve Early, and Ross McIntire to Fort Benning, forty miles south of Warm Springs.

The first postmortem cover-up began even before McIntire left for Georgia. "The president's blood pressure was all right and had been for some time, and there was absolutely no apparent cause for the stroke," McIntire told Stettinius.[9] He told Ambassador Joseph E. Davies that in trying to slim down, Franklin had gone from 190 pounds to 160, but too abruptly, blaming unnamed "others" for convincing the president to keep dieting when he really wanted to gain weight.[10]

Even at such a trying moment, Eleanor's compassion shone through. Remembering that her friend Elinor Morgenthau was recovering from a heart attack in Florida and fearing that the news of Franklin's death might cause a setback, she asked her private secretary to call the Morgenthau home and tell the nurse to turn off the radio in the sickroom.

Less than a year into his second term, Franklin had left detailed instructions how he wanted his passing handled should he die in office.[11] He composed a memorandum, dated December 26, 1937, to his eldest son, James, sealed it in an envelope, and placed it in his personal safe.[12] The document reveals Franklin's awareness of his fatal prognosis in 1937 and his desire to assure the diagnosis should remain secret forever. It stipulated that "the casket be of absolute simplicity, dark wood, that the body be not embalmed nor hermetically sealed and that the grave not be lined with brick, cement or stones." Tellingly, he named the Reverend Endicott Peabody, twenty-four years his senior, to conduct the funeral service.[13]

---

9 Campbell, T.M., Herring, G.C., *The Diaries of Edward R. Stettinius, Jr: 1943-1945*, 316, As quoted in Ferrell, Robert H. *The Dying President*, 12.
10 *Ibid.*, 12–13.
11 Asbell, *When F.D.R. Died*, 19.
12 Roosevelt and Shalett, 366.
13 Asbell, *When F.D.R. Died*, 198.

Eleanor found the envelope soon after her husband's death, but kept it unopened until she could give it to James, who did not return from his military posting in the Philippines until after the funeral. Owing to that delay, several of Franklin's wishes were not carried out. One was his interdiction on embalming.

With Dr. Paullin's help, Bruenn engaged the services of an Atlanta mortuary, H. Patterson & Co. Paullin later wrote that Polly Delano told him of her cousin's wishes not to be embalmed but Eleanor vetoed that dictate.[14]

The subject of choosing a casket had come up while those assembled at the Little White House were awaiting Eleanor's arrival. Grace Tully recalled that Franklin had selected a solid mahogany casket with a copper lining for his mother. Hassett reminded the group the coffin had to accommodate a six foot-three-inch body.

At 5:47 p.m. Eastern time, the International News Service tapped out one of the shortest news flashes in history: "FDR DEAD." Within two minutes all nationwide broadcasting systems interrupted their programming with a similar announcement.[15] Hearing the news on his car radio en route to the Little White House, neurosurgeon Swanson turned back to Atlanta.[16]

Four hours after leaving Franklin, Lucy Rutherfurd and her companions were passing through Macon, Georgia. Desperate for news, Lucy asked to stop at the Dempsey Hotel and to call the Little White House. Unable to get through by pay phone, Shoumatoff saw hotel employees crying and overheard them talking about the president's death. The trio resumed their journey with Lucy sobbing in the back seat. Robbins became aware of the reason for their sudden departure from Warm Springs only when he heard it on the radio.[17] Flags were already flying at half-staff. The threesome took a wrong turn and did not reach the Rutherfurd estate until after midnight.[18]

McIntire, Early, and Eleanor arrived at the Little White House at 11 p.m. McIntire went into conference with Bruenn and Paullin while Early spoke with Bill Hassett about the crush of reporters expected to arrive in the morning.

---

14 Goldsmith, 174.
15 Asbell. *When F.D.R. Died,* 79.
16 Personal communication with Dr. Hal "Toby" Raper.
17 Shoumatoff, 121.
18 *Ibid.*

Eleanor was the calmest person in the room. After hugging a tearful Grace Tully, Polly, and Daisy, she asked each in turn what had happened. Tully was almost too emotional to speak. Daisy calmly related the details of Franklin's collapse. Then Polly dropped a bomb, telling Eleanor that Franklin had been sitting for a portrait by a friend of Lucy Rutherfurd and that Lucy had been there as well, staying in the guest cottage.[19]

Eleanor asked "for a minute" to be alone with her husband. She stayed five. When she emerged from the bedroom, Polly continued her vindictive barrage, revealing that not only had Lucy been at Warm Springs, but that she had been seeing Franklin for years, even at the White House where Anna acted as hostess. Eleanor internalized her emotions and played out the mirage of her marriage for the sake of her family—and her country.

No one present was aware of Franklin's stipulation about his coffin, so a solid brass and copper model was selected from the two brought by Patterson. Embalming began at 12:33 a.m. on Friday, April 13.[20] Mortician F. Haden Snoderly described the corpse. "Rigor mortis had set in, since nine hours had elapsed since time of death," he wrote. "Discoloration was very evident about the face and hands. Numerous skin blisters all over the body [likely caused by an allergy to the penicillin]. Apparently he had lost considerable weight. There

---

19 Laura Franklin Delano was FDR's first cousin. Her father, Warren, was Franklin's mother Sara's brother and president of the Delano Coal Company, one of the largest in Pennsylvania. Her mother, Jennie Walters, was the great-granddaughter of the world's richest man, John Jacob Astor. As a child Laura disdained all drink other than Apollinaris Mineral Water and thus acquired the nickname "Polly." Her life was devoted to the avocations of the idle rich—breeding Irish Setters and dachshunds and for many years judging dog shows in the United States and abroad. An accomplished carriage driver, she won numerous awards at the annual Dutchess County Fair, driving the horses raised at her father's vast estate, Steen Valetje, in nearby Barrytown-on-Hudson and those of her cousin and Hudson Valley neighbor, Helen Astor. She was also an active member of the Walters Art Gallery in Baltimore that had been founded by her maternal grandfather, Henry Walters, a railroad magnate, consummate collector, and founder of the Walters Art Museum in Baltimore. Naturally flamboyant, Polly adopted the peculiar style of an overabundant display of jewelry and purple-dyed hair. The sharply accented widow's peak she carefully applied to her forehead each morning became her trademark. While Polly could be kind and compassionate, she shared FDR's mother's and Theodore's daughter Alice's disdain for Eleanor. As biographer Jim Bishop wrote "There are 'Eleanor people' and there are 'Franklin' people, and the contempt each reserves for the other is unremitting." (*FDR's Last Year,* xi.). Polly was most definitely in the Franklin camp.
20 Franklin was triskaidekaphobic and made a point of avoiding travel on Friday the thirteenth. Ironically, his last journey began on that day.

was heavy puffing under the eyes. Naturally, his limbs were not normal. His abdomen was noticeably distended."[21]

The distended abdomen—a condition that preceded death—is consistent with a bowel obstruction from metastatic cancer from the frequent small feedings that had dammed up in Franklin's blocked intestines. Snoderly and his colleagues had great difficulty injecting embalming fluid into Franklin's "sclerotic" arteries—confirming the presence of severe arteriosclerosis from smoking, a fatty diet, and hypertension.

At 9:15 a.m., the six-hundred-pound casket containing Franklin's embalmed remains was moved into a hearse. To the plaintive sound of drumbeats, a color guard, a band, and about 3,000 soldiers preceded the casket on a thirty-six-minute journey to the train station. The cortege made a brief stop in front of Georgia Hall, where Navy Chief Petty Officer Graham Jackson, tears streaming down his face, played one of Franklin's favorite hymns, "Going Home," on his accordion.[22]

Overnight, a team of rail workers and carpenters had transformed the press car into a catafalque, allowing onlookers to view Franklin's flag-draped coffin as the train rolled north.[23] By the time it reached Washington, 400,000 mourners were waiting to see it pass through the streets of the capital.[24]

---

21 Undated memorandum, author's collection, courtesy of Phillis (Oliver) Abbott.

22 Asbell, *When F.D.R. Died*, 134.

23 Any information one could possibly want to know about the preparations for the funeral train has been presented by Robert Klara in his painstakingly researched book, *FDR's Funeral Train*, St. Martin's Press, 2010.

24 Since Bill Hassett had identified "Nicholas Robbins" as the artist who was painting Roosevelt when he was stricken in Warm Springs, a gaggle of reporters was waiting outside his Manhattan apartment when he and Madame Shoumatoff pulled up after a two-day trip up U.S. 1. The artist wanted no part of it. After a mad chase through Harlem, they shook their pursuers on the Triborough Bridge, finally arriving at the home of Madame Shoumatoff's daughter in Locust Valley on Long Island. Despite orders from Steve Early to the contrary, after a call to Aiken, a press conference was arranged for the next morning at 10 a.m. The artist confirmed her presence at the Little White House but was successful in not revealing the presence of Lucy (Shoumatoff, p. 124). Other than for family members, close friends, and the staff at Warm Springs, the secret would be protected until after Lucy's death in 1948 when Walter Trohan was tipped off by Mike Reilly to her presence, but the publisher of the *Chicago Tribune*, "Colonel" Robert McCormick, refused to use the information. (While McCormick ran a distinctly anti-Roosevelt newspaper, he was also an alumnus, as FDR, of Groton School.) The public did not become widely aware of the FDR/Lucy affair until Jonathan Daniels' cover story in the September 2, 1966, issue of *Life* magazine, nearly four years after Eleanor's death.

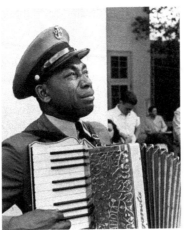

Graham Jackson at FDRs funeral procession, Warm Springs, April 13, 1945.

Robert Sherwood epitomized the reactions of Franklin's staff and close associates. "I couldn't believe it when somebody told me he was dead," Sherwood said. "Like everybody else, I listened and listened to the radio, waiting for the announcement—probably in his own gaily reassuring voice—that it had all been a big mistake, that the banking crisis and the war were over and everything was going to be 'fine—grand—perfectly bully.' But when the realization finally did get through all I could think of was, 'It finally crushed him. He couldn't stand up under it any longer' ... The fears and hopes of hundreds of millions of human beings throughout the world had been bearing down on the mind of one man, until the pressure was more than mortal tissue could withstand."[25] A memorial service was conducted in the White House East Room. The benediction was given at 4:33 p.m. That evening Eleanor returned alone. She asked for the casket to be opened, put a few flowers in, placed her wedding ring on Franklin's hand, then ordered it sealed.[26]

Franklin never got the wish he expressed in his 1937 memorandum to rest for a night in front of the fireplace in Springwood's "big room," nor was his memorial service conducted at St. James Church. A team of horses pulled the caisson holding Franklin's casket up a path lined by ranks of soldiers to the

---

25 Sherwood, 680.
26 Asbell, *When FDR Died*, 183.

final resting place he had always wanted—in his mother's rose garden where the sundial stood.

An honor guard standing at attention lined the hemlock hedge surrounding the garden. At 10 a.m. on April 15, the opening salvo of a twenty-one-gun salute was fired on the grounds of the library to the east. Fala barked in response to each round.[27] The stocky 78-year-old Reverend George W. Anthony, rector of the St. James Episcopal church, stood at the head of the grave for the ten-minute service. Facing him were Eleanor, flanked by her son, Brigadier General Elliott Roosevelt, on her left, and her daughter Anna, with her husband, Colonel John Boettiger, on her right. Behind them were Eleanor's four daughters-in-law, in the next row were President and Mrs. Harry Truman. A delegation from the Senate and House stood with members of the Supreme Court and Cabinet on the west; White House staff and other dignitaries on the east.

The New York Times broke its self-enforced silence about Franklin's declining health on April 13. "The condition of the health of President Roosevelt raised doubts in the minds of those in the capital who have had regular contact with him over the last two years, largely because official statements regarding it appeared to be in conflict with visible evidence of his physical condition," the paper wrote.[28] Walter Trohan's detailed account of Franklin's deterioration, including mention of prostate cancer, appeared on the front page of the *Chicago Tribune*. The article reported that "Howard Gerald Bruenn, a New York City heart specialist was commissioned in the navy in late 1942 and assigned to the President." The impact was virtually nil. Another obvious Trohan production was an unbylined three-part series headlined "The Strange Death of Franklin D. Roosevelt" in *News Story* magazine, beginning in June 1945.[29] The series provided previously unreported details about Franklin's prostate cancer, his collapse in Hyde Park on Palm Sunday, and the strict press censorship. Unsubstantiated scuttlebutt about Franklin's health fell on deaf ears.

27 This comes from an intimate and stirring account of the funeral by Eleanor's friend Trude Lash in a letter to her husband on April 15th. Lash, Joseph, 84.

28 "Roosevelt Health Long Under Doubt." *New York Times*, April 13,1945.

29 *News Story Magazine*, edited and published by Herbert Moore, New York, Volume 3, numbers 3–5, June-October 1945.

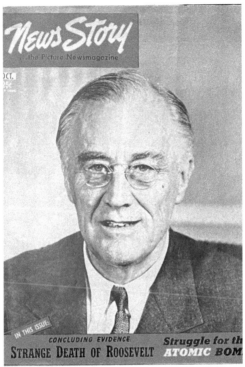

Cover of News Story magazine, October 1945

Franklin's death certificate, signed on April 13 by Howard Bruenn, gave the primary cause of death as cerebral hemorrhage. Only one contributing cause was listed—arteriosclerosis. The postmortem cover-up had begun in earnest.

■ Chapter 29
■ Burnishing an Image

In 1946, publishing house G.P. Putnam's Sons brought out Ross McIntire's memoir, *White House Physician*. Co-author George Creel had been Woodrow Wilson's propaganda czar during World War I.[1] The book lacks an index or photographs. Short on facts, the project was nearly aborted over Creel's frustration with McIntire's reluctance to provide substantive information.[2]

White House Physician is a repository of outrageous falsehoods. McIntire claimed, for instance, that Franklin had neither high blood pressure nor arteriosclerosis. "President Roosevelt did not have either of these. His blood pressure was not alarming at any time," McIntire wrote. "In fact, on the morning of the day he died it was well within normal limits for a man of his age."[3,4]

During preparation for his memoir, McIntire asked Howard Bruenn and James Paullin to provide recollections of their interactions with Franklin. The doctors gave him what he wanted: "During the last six weeks of his life, his trend of thoughts, his appraisal of situations and his evaluations of circumstances were just as clear and contemporaneous and he maintained his superiority until the end," Bruenn wrote. He also included a statement he would later contradict: "As you know, it was my good fortune to be with the President for almost *two years* (emphasis added) before he died."[5] Paullin also responded with less than complete candor. "It was thought that [Franklin] had a moderate degree of arteriosclerosis with a variable hypertension, some electrocardiographic evidence of coronary artery disease, some cloudiness in his sinuses and some evidence [of] a recent attack of influenza," the Atlanta internist wrote of his alleged first encounter with Franklin on April 2, 1944. Of their meeting in July, Paullin wrote that the president "was most jovial ... we talked to him at

---

1 It is indicative of the intent of the book that McIntire was assisted in the writing of it by George Creel, who had been the head of the United States Committee on Public Information, a propaganda organization created by President Woodrow Wilson during World War I.

2 Ross McIntire files. FDRL.

3 McIntire, 239.

4 The last readings that survive, taken less than a week before his death, ranged from a high 170/88 to an alarming 240/130.

5 Goldsmith, 104.

least an hour or longer and at that time I stressed upon him the importance of moderation in all things." Paullin neglected to mention that this was the time when he, McIntire, and Frank Lahey had informed the president they did not believe he would survive another term.

When Anna Halsted moved into the White House in December 1943, the only restriction imposed on her was a ban on keeping a diary. She was schooled in the art of cover-up at Yalta. "I have found out through Bruenn who won't let me tell Ross [McIntire] I know, that this ticker situation is far more serious than I ever knew," she wrote to her husband, "and the biggest difficulty in handling the situation here is that we can of course tell no one of the ticker troubles (Better tear off and destroy this paragraph.)."[6]

As time went on, Anna became even more protective of her father. "It is becoming increasingly clear that [Anna] means to be what the papers are suggesting that she is—a sort of special secretary close to the President, handling details for him and serving as intermediary for others who handle details for him," Jonathan Daniels wrote. "She had been greatly concerned about the strains on her father ... Howard Bruenn had told her he must greatly restrict his activities. So she had a plan. The President should see very few people. In so far as possible I was to see those who wished to see him, and then pass on the matters presented to me to Anna and her husband for decision without burdening the President with any but the greatest matters.

I knew that no such plan could possibly work. It would have amounted only to something like the almost regency which Mrs. Wilson and Cary Grayson had assumed out of necessity during the former President's illness."[7]

"The tragic theme of restricted access, sanctioned by a physician and exercised by a closely positioned woman, inflicted itself once again upon the office of the American presidency," neurosurgeon Bert Park wrote decades later in his book about the impact of health on world leaders. "[Even] if Anna's impact on events was arguably less than was Edith Wilson's, one cannot avoid a disquieting sense of déjà vu. Daniels's description so closely parallels what had occurred twenty-five years earlier that the names Grayson, [personal secretary Joseph P.] Tumulty[8] and Edith might almost be interchanged with

---

6 Anna Roosevelt Boettinger to John Boettinger, February 4, 1945, Anna Roosevelt Halsted papers, FDRL.
7 Daniels, 265–266.
8 Joseph Patrick Tumulty was Woodrow Wilson's private secretary during his Governorship

McIntire, Daniels and Anna."[9] After her father's death, Anna took on the role of Roosevelt family watchdog—on alert for anything she felt might stain his legacy.

The Twenty-Second Amendment to the Constitution, which limits a president to two four-year terms, was passed by a two-thirds majority of Congress on March 21, 1947. John F. Kennedy, then a freshman congressman, voted in favor. That a Democrat from a northern state would cast a seemingly anti-Roosevelt vote caused an interlocutor to ask Kennedy about it. Kennedy said that two months after Franklin's death, he had spoken with Frank Lahey, who told him the late president's doctors should have warned him not to run again.[10] Lahey apparently hadn't informed Kennedy that he was one of those doctors.

In 1948, Dr. Emanuel Josephson, a fifty-year-old eye specialist, self-published a potpourri of wild conspiracy theories under the provocative title *The Strange Death of Franklin Roosevelt*. Among Josephson's allegations were that Franklin may have died of suicide, murder, or arsenic poisoning and that he had been replaced by a body double. Amid all the nonsense, Josephson also wrote, "It takes no great medical skill to diagnose the character of the growth over President Roosevelt's left eyebrow. It had the characteristic appearance and behavior of a mole turned malignant and rapidly growing, a type of cancer, known as melanosarcoma ... one of the most malignant forms of cancer."[11] No one gave Josephson any credence, but his book left a lasting impression on Anna as an example of how easily her father's image could be denigrated.[12]

Anna divorced John Boettinger in December 1948 and returned to her career in journalism as editor of *The Woman's Digest*. Boettinger remarried in November 1949, took an unsatisfying job in Holland, then jumped seven stories to his death out of a New York City hotel room on Halloween 1950.

---

of New Jersey and both terms of his presidency. He did much of his work after his devastating stroke.

9 Park, B.E., *The Impact of Illness on World Leaders*. University of Pennsylvania Press, 1986, 262.

10 The conversation occurred at the time JFK was recuperating from back surgery by Lahey Clinic surgeon James Poppen. Poppen remained the Kennedy family's neurosurgeon. He was summoned to Los Angeles to operate on Robert Kennedy after he was shot in the head on Sirhan Sirhan in June 1968.

11 Josephson, E., *The Strange Death of Franklin D. Roosevelt*, 236–237 PUB INFO.

12 Lomazow and Fettmann, 195.

The first serious challenge to the first postmortem cover-up came on February 15, 1949, when "The Truth About FDR's Health," by Minnesota physician Karl Christian Wold, was featured in the widely circulated, highly reputable *Look* magazine.[13] Wold asserted that, starting as early as 1938, Franklin had suffered a series of four strokes.[14] The first allegedly occurred in late summer 1938 while Franklin was visiting his son James at the Mayo Clinic. "Recovery from the hemorrhage was quick and complete," Wold wrote. No corroboration was given.[15] The doctor claimed a second stroke occurred in December 1943, also without offering any solid evidence, though a stroke at this juncture was within the realm of probability. The third stroke supposedly occurred on March 25, 1945. This was a misdiagnosis of Franklin's real and disturbing grand mal seizure. The fourth was the fatal cerebral hemorrhage on April 12. Wold's unnamed source was Walter Trohan, who had laid out the identical timeline in the *Tribune* two months after Franklin's death.[16,17]

McIntire labeled Wold's claims "completely erroneous," telling the Washington *Times*, "if they are interested in facts, they should have checked with me first."[18] Anna wrote a lengthy rebuttal in the May 1949 issue of *The Women's Digest* and Elliott skewered Wold in *Liberty* the same month, while also exposing Trohan as the source of the story.[19] *Time* labeled Trohan the "topflight hatchet man of the *Chicago Tribune* in its account of the controversy."[20]

The issue of Franklin's health came up again in 1951 in a letter to *The New York Times* from former Democratic Party chairman James A. Farley. "We saw tragically in the case of President Roosevelt an utter breakdown of his great strength in his third term," Farley wrote. "Worse, we saw his nomination in 1944 when it was widely known among political leaders that he was a dying man."[21]

---

13 The article was excerpted from Wold's book "Mr. President—How Is Your Health?"
14 "The Truth About Roosevelt's Health. Year by Year." *Look*, February 15, 1949, 23.
15 Trohan also vaguely mentioned "a heart condition which, it was feared, might become grave." in a 1947 article.
16 "Reveal Stroke Almost Killed FDR on March 25," *Chicago Tribune*, June 24, 1945.
17 Wold admitted to Elliott Roosevelt in a telephone call that Trohan was his source. Hansen, R., *The Year We Had No President*. Lincoln, NE: University of Nebraska Press, 1962, 59.
18 Roosevelt Suffered 4 Strokes, First in '38, Physician Says." *Washington Evening Star*, February 4, 1949, 18.
19 Roosevelt, E., "They're Lying About F.D.R.'s Health." *Liberty*, April 26, 19.
20 "Counter Fire," *Time*, May 2, 1949.
21 *New York Times*, August 5, 1951.

Those last five words set Ross McIntire off—though many newspapers in the days following Franklin's death had pretty much said the same thing. But Farley was the first former member of Franklin's inner circle to make such a claim. McIntire responded with a letter to the *Washington Star*, which had published an editorial agreeing with Farley. His protest hardly constituted a denial. Farley's letter, McIntire charged, was an attack on the "excellent doctors who worked with me and whose reputations cannot be challenged." Besides, McIntire wrote, Farley hadn't seen the president "for a period of several years," so "it could not have been his personal observation that the president was a dying man." McIntire also wrote that Franklin knew his own physical condition at all times—which, though true, evaded the question of what that condition actually was.[22]

McIntire's other parry to the Farley kerfuffle was to give an interview to *U.S. News & World Report*, which ran in the magazine's March 22, 1951, issue under the headline "Did the U.S. Elect a Dying President?" His comments were little more than an expansion of the story he had told five years earlier in *White House Physician*.

Much of the press let McIntire's interview speak for itself. One exception, the Hearst-owned Boston *Herald*, ran an editorial saying the paper was "not the least bit surprised" McIntire had "denied what Dr. Wold reported" because "not to have denied it would have made him a liar." After all, the *Herald* wrote, "Many leading specialists throughout the country who never had the opportunity of examining the President had ample basis for dire diagnosis from his declining physical appearance. These external symptoms were particularly noticeable to the correspondents, even though they lacked the medical competence to judge their meaning. They long suspected something on the order of what Dr. Wold reports."[23]

Eleanor Roosevelt held her tongue about her husband's health until an interview with Clayton Knowles in *The New York Times* on August 9, 1956.[24] Her husband's physicians had told him in the summer of 1944 that Franklin "could quite easily go on with the activities of the presidency," Eleanor told Knowles,

---

22 *Washington Star*, March 10, 1951. As quoted in *Lomazow and Fettmann*, 199.
23 *Boston Herald*, September 30, 1951. erAlHH.
24 Knowles, C., "Wife Says Doctors Cleared Roosevelt," *New York Times* August 9, 1956.

at the same time insisting that health played no role in his decision to run. "He never gave his health much thought," she said, "and neither did any of us."[25]

Eleanor's statements fly in the face of every available piece of evidence. Her mother-daughter correspondence with Anna is testimony to the extent to which Franklin's condition disturbed the Roosevelt women. Daisy Suckley's diary repeatedly confirms how much attention Franklin paid his health. But none of this was publicly known, so Eleanor was able to parrot without challenge the fabulist line of a martyr president who persevered with complete disregard for his physical well-being—not that there was really anything noticeably wrong with him, anyway. This remained Eleanor's stance until she died on November 7, 1962 after months of ill health due to what was only diagnosed postmortem as a rare form of tuberculosis.

---

25 *New York Times,* August 9, 1956.

■ Chapter 30
■ Manufacturing a Lie

Since 1930, Franklin had been diagnosed with two cancers, subjected to a series of cosmetic surgeries, and had made dozens of visits to his medical sanctuaries at Warm Springs and Bethesda.[1] In 1934, he had nearly died from acute hemorrhage. During the run-up to his third nomination in 1940, he was out of the public eye for weeks at a time while undergoing medical treatment and, in 1941, had endured months of life-threatening intestinal bleeding. All the while, Ross McIntire and Stephen Early had been masterminding a campaign to hide his maladies.

A well-researched scholarly study written by historian Herman E. Bateman in 1956 provides a comprehensive assessment of Franklin's health from 1942 through 1945. The paper is an accurate measure of what was known—and what was not known—eleven years after his death.

"Observations on President Roosevelt's Health during World War II"[2] presented a plethora of opinions on both sides of the spectrum about Franklin's physical fitness. Bateman frequently cited the rosy viewpoint by Ross McIntire in his memoir and public statements, but did not denigrate his reputation—McIntire did not die until three years later. On the other hand, Bateman referred to a book by FDR's bête noire, John T. Flynn, that alleged McIntire had "foisted a 'hopeless invalid' upon an unsuspecting country in the 1944 election."[3] The paper makes little mention of preexisting illness other than polio, says nothing about cardiovascular disease, and very little about cognitive problems. There is no reference to cancer.

Bateman concluded his 20-page paper by saying, "Like the accounts in the newspapers, those contained in the various memoirs—with the prominent exception of McIntire's book—devoted relatively little space to questions about the President's health. But they differ from the newspapers in one important

---

1 Crispell, K.R., Gomez, C., *Hidden Illness in the White House,* 118. States "Roosevelt visited [Bethesda] incognito at least twenty-nine times from 1941 to 1945."
2 Bateman, H.E., "Observations on President Roosevelt's Health during World War II." *Mississippi Valley Historical Review* June, 1956;43(1):82–102.
3 Flynn, 412.

respect: usually more space was allotted or at least more concern shown about the subject in the time after the November election then before it. The proportioning of space in the memoirs reflects more accurately then the newspapers the worsening of the President's health, though their accuracy may have been partly the wisdom of hindsight. Understandably, too, the associates who may have felt disquiet before the election would not be eager to publish it. But granting this and the number of other reservations, the evidence to date shows only partial signs or traces of a deteriorated physical condition at the most critical time, the election of 1944. Only an omniscient observer could have forecast the succeeding events with certainty." The paper makes it crystal clear that McIntire and Early's cover-ups were wildly successful.

James Paullin passed away of a heart attack in 1951 while examining a patient in his Atlanta office.[4] Frank Lahey succumbed in Boston in 1953 in the midst of performing an operation. After Ross McIntire suffered a fatal heart attack in 1959, the only physician left to oversee the cover-up of Franklin's health was Howard Bruenn.

In 1962, Franklin's former medical aide, George Fox, had thoughts about writing a book, but expressed reservations about "opening the bedroom door a little too wide."[5] The potential exposé was likely squelched after news of Fox's intention reached Bruenn.

Despite the rebuttals of Anna and Elliott, Dr. Wold's allegations in *Look* continued to percolate.[6] The Roosevelt family remained silent until an article by Dr. John D. Ratliff, "How Science is Saving Stroke Victims," appeared in the March 1962 issue of *Today's Health*, a general-interest magazine published by the American Medical Association. Ratliff echoed Wold's assertion that "Franklin D. Roosevelt had five minor strokes before the final catastrophe which killed him."[7]

The magazine agreed to publish a rejoinder in its December issue by Dr. James A. Halsted, a Harvard-educated internist who had married Anna Roosevelt in 1952 and assumed the role of Roosevelt family medical

4 *New York Times*, August 5, 1951.
5 Rigdon papers, Georgia Southern University.
6 References to strokes appeared in a book by Marx, R., *Health of the Presidents*. New York: GP Putnams, 1960, and an article by McConnell, B.H. , "The Little Stroke. A Report on 89 Cases." *Journal of the American Geriatric Society* February 9 1961; 110–118; Lomazow and Fettmann, 204.
7 Ratliff, J.D., "How Science is Saving Stroke Victims." *Today's Health*, March 1942.

spokesman. Halsted wrote in "FDR's Little Strokes, a Medical Myth," that his wife had told him she "never saw the slightest sign of 'little strokes' in the year and a half she was her father's personal assistant"—notwithstanding what Anna had told Dr. Louis Schmidt about Franklin's "little hemorrhages" in 1947 and Colonel McCormick about his "amnesia" in 1948.

Halsted invoked a surprising source for support. "Presumably [Ratliff] did not read Dr. McIntire's book, otherwise he must have been willing to assume that Dr. McIntire, a vice-admiral in the United States Navy, who was in nearly daily attendance upon the President from 1933 to 1945, did not tell the truth."

Halsted's article set the stage for a new postmortem cover-up, far more daring than the previous one. "It is important to get at the truth in order to set the record straight," Halsted wrote. "Otherwise this myth would lend credence to the assumption that Roosevelt's judgement was seriously impaired by his supposed ill-health. Going on unchallenged, it might become part of a documented 'history' in the years to come."

Anna Halsted's earliest known communication with Howard Bruenn after her father's death was in 1963, when she advised him against donating his papers to the FDR Library unless he restricted access to them "for a considerable period yet to come."[8] In 1967, Anna was asked for an interview by journalist Roul Tunley, who was in negotiations with publisher G.P. Putnam's Sons to write a book about the last years of her father's life. Anna declined, telling Tunley it was her "deep hope" that Howard Bruenn would soon be writing a paper about her father's health in a medical journal.[9] Lacking input from the president's family, Tunley cancelled his project.

Unbeknownst to Anna, on April 11, 1956, Eleanor had written to surgeon general of the Navy[10] Rear Admiral Bartholomew W. Hogan, to request her husband's medical records.[11] When none were found at Bethesda, Hogan went to Ross McIntire, who said he had only a few laboratory reports that he had forwarded to Eleanor. Many were from the time of Franklin's severe anemia in 1941, an episode Eleanor already had been told of in detail by McIntire. Eleanor sent the records to the FDR Library and dropped the matter.

---

8 Anna Roosevelt Halsted to Howard G. Bruenn, March 5, 1963, Anna Roosevelt Halsted papers, FDRL-HP.
9 Anna Halsted to Bruenn, July 14, 1967, Bruenn papers, FDRL.
10 Official military file of Franklin D. Roosevelt, National archives.
11 The original plan was to publish the article in the *Journal of Medical Biography*.

With Bruenn's medical paper in mind, Anna started a search of her own, also contacting the Navy surgeon general, then Vice Admiral Robert B. Brown.

"Mrs Halstead [sic] called and told a thorough search made and no records found," the Navy replied on July 6, 1967. "Doubtful that any were kept by Navy since President Roosevelt was never hospitalized at Bethesda.

"Mrs. Halsted said Mrs. Ross McIntire told Mrs. Roosevelt that Admiral McIntire destroyed the records.

"A Dr. Howard Bruenn, formerly in the Navy and stationed at the White House, is writing a short article on President Roosevelt's health in his later years from personal memory and notes he kept. This will be published in a medical historical journal and has the blessing of the Roosevelt family."

When Anna learned about the laboratory reports her mother had obtained, she pronounced herself mystified as to "why mother never requested the medical records until 1957 [actually, 1956]; and I wonder what prompted her at that time."

After Bruenn had met with the Halsteds to plan the medical paper,[12] Anna wrote him on July 14, 1967, telling Bruenn that her husband was going to go to the FDR Library to review her father's medical records and would send him his analysis.[13] Dr. Halsted's letter to Bruenn on August 18 included mention of the 1941 transfusion that the cardiologist later denied knowing of.[14]

The Halsted/Bruenn project took on increased urgency in late 1969 after a book published in London, set for American release on New Year's Day 1970, alleged Roosevelt's terminal illness was due to "malignant deposits from a pigmented growth." In *The Pathology of Leadership*,[15] British physician/historian Hugh L'Etang, wrote that an "American physician" had "noticed that a pigmented naevus [mole] above Roosevelt's left eyebrow did not appear in photographs after 1943" and it had been removed surgically.[16] Alarmed by

---

12 The exact date of this meeting is unknown.
13 Anna Roosevelt Halsted to Howard G. Bruenn, July 14, 1967, Anna Roosevelt Halsted papers, FDRL.
14 Howard Bruenn papers, FDRL.
15 L'Etang, H., *The Pathology of Leadership*. London: Heineman Medical Books Ltd., 1969, 95.
16 The physician was most probably F.M. Massie. Massie was a surgeon who had published a paper in 1961 in which he commented on FDR's pigmented lesion and its eventual

L'Etang's eagle-eyed research, Anna wrote to three of her four brothers on November 5, 1969—she and Elliott were not speaking—informing them about Bruenn's paper and asking their consent to publish it in *Annals of Internal Medicine* at the twenty-fifth anniversary of their father's death. L'Etang's book, Anna told her brothers, had made an "unequivocal statement that father was killed by a brain tumor ... Dr. Bruenn's present hope is that his article might appear in print either before or at approximately the same time as Dr. L'Etang's book."[17] After receiving positive responses, Anna sent a letter to the journal's editor with the family's endorsement of Bruenn's submission.[18]

Twenty years after Franklin's death, No one outside Franklin's innermost circle had any inkling of his medical problems during the last eighteen months of his life. By coincidence, historian James MacGregor Burns was working on *Soldier of Freedom*, a sequel to his best-selling 1956 biography of Franklin, *The Lion and the Fox*, and reached out to Anna for her help to arrange an interview with Dr. Bruenn. Sensing opportunity, Anna embraced the overture and set up a line of communications between the historian and the physician. Having no reason to doubt the credibility of the firsthand information he was getting, Burns enthusiastically incorporated Bruenn and the Halsteds' carefully couched, well-rehearsed language into his manuscript.[19]

On January 3, 1970, Burns wrote to Bruenn to inform him that the release of *Soldier of Freedom* had been delayed and he would be writing a magazine article to appear contemporaneously with publication of the medical paper. That article ran as the feature story in the April 11, 1970, *Saturday Review*. "Bruenn's disclosures, which are as full and authoritative as anything we are likely to have on the matter, will force us to revise most interpretations of the significance of Roosevelt's medical condition during his final year," Burns wrote.[20] This was surely music to the ears of the three co-conspirators. *Soldier of Freedom* won the Pulitzer Prize for history in 1971 and became the source for all subsequent biographies with respect to Franklin's health during the last years of his life.

---

disappearance, concluding that it was a malignant melanoma based on a slide from Walter Reed Army Hospital taken from Roosevelt's body during postmortem. As it turns out, the slide was later shown to be from a 27-year-old sailor. Franklin's remains were never autopsied.

17 Bruenn papers, FDRL.

18 *Ibid.*

19 The correspondence between the Halsteds, Bruenn, Burns, and the editors of *Annals of Internal Medicine* is discussed in chapter 15 of *FDR's Deadly Secret*.

20 "FDR: The Untold Story of His Last Year." *Saturday Review*, April 11, 1970, 12.

The Bruenn/Halsted collaboration came to fruition when "Clinical Notes on the Illness and Death of President Franklin D. Roosevelt" appeared in the April 1970 issue of *Annals of Internal Medicine*.[21] Bruenn was credited as the sole author. Despite considerable contextual and editorial input from the Halsteds, the couple chose to remain in the background.

"Clinical Notes" perverts the truth with false narratives and purposeful omissions. More than a mere cover-up of Franklin's medical problems, the paper rewrites history to exclude their occurrence. An editorial published with the article lays out its two most important purposes. "The speculation in a recently published book (based on the showing of an unlabeled slide from Walter Reed Hospital) that the President was suffering from a metastatic melanoma in the brain, is laid to rest by Dr. Bruenn; there was no clinical evidence for such a lesion, and no autopsy was performed," the editors wrote. "We are given, by Dr. Bruenn, the picture of a great and gallant man, fatigued by the burdens of his office and by his hypertension and reduced cardiac reserve, yet quite able to exercise his judgment and to use the fruits of his unique knowledge and experience in guiding the war effort."[22]

"Clinical Notes" claims or implies that:

- Unsatisfied with her father's medical care, Anna asked Dr. McIntire for a second opinion.
- Franklin was not diagnosed with any serious chronic health problem (other than polio) until he was examined for the first time by Dr. Bruenn on March 27, 1944 (actually, March 28) and that problem was exclusively cardiac.
- His weight loss was due to a self-enforced diet.
- There was never any malignancy.
- There were never any cognitive difficulties.

All of these assertions are false. The scope of the deception is astounding.

Though the *Annals of Internal Medicine* editorial specifically denied Franklin had a brain tumor, no mention of malignancy appears in the paper. Henceforth, the word "cancer" disappeared from Bruenn's vocabulary. Asked in 1990 by

---

21 Bruenn, H.G., "Clinical Notes on the Illness and Death of President Franklin D. Roosevelt." Annals of Internal Medicine 1970 April;72(4):579–91.

22 Editorial board, *American Journal of Medicine*, April 1970.

Naval Medical Historian Jan Kenneth Herman about the pigmented lesion above Franklin's left eye, Bruenn replied, "That's a photographic error or something. He never had anything wrong with that."[23]

"Clinical Notes" begins with a statement which empowers Bruenn and the Halsteds to say anything they want with no ability for corroboration. "The original hospital chart in which all clinical progress notes as well as the results of the various laboratory tests were incorporated was kept in the safe at the U.S. Naval Hospital, Bethesda, Md.," Bruenn wrote. "After the President's death this chart could not be found."

The "original hospital chart" indeed included progress notes and laboratory reports—using dozens of aliases Franklin had been assigned over the years. This is why biographers had difficulty finding it—until two doctors did. In 1981, Kenneth R. Crispell, emeritus professor of medicine and law at the University of Virginia, and his medical student, Carlos F. Gomez, filed a Freedom of Information Act (FOIA) request to the National Naval Medical Center for Franklin's medical records in conjunction with researching their book, *Hidden Illness in the White House*. The response from chief legal officer revealed that Franklin had visited the hospital twenty-nine times between 1941 and 1945 under a variety of aliases,[24] some of which are identical to those used in the medical records Eleanor obtained in 1956—proof that Franklin's medical records existed as late as 1981. The present location of the file is unknown.

The second paragraph of "Clinical Notes" flatly asserts, "I first saw President Roosevelt professionally in March 1944." But on August 1, 1946, he had written McIntire, "As you know, it was my good fortune to be with the President for almost two years before he died."[25] Furthermore, in 1951 McIntire told *U.S. News and World Report* "In the last couple of years I used Howard as I had used Dr. Duncan before him."

The duration of Bruenn's service as Franklin's cardiologist became a secret only after the false narrative was hatched in 1970. The day after Franklin died, Walter Trohan's front page *Chicago Tribune* article said, "Howard Gerald

23 Herman interview of Bruenn at his home in Riverdale (Bronx) New York, January 31, 1990. Text courtesy of Jan Herman.
24 FOIA request, 81-DFI-1259. Crispell, K., Gomez, C., *Hidden Illness in the White House*. Durham and London: Duke University Press, 1988, Chapter 3, footnote 79.
25 Bruenn to McIntire, August 1, 1946. McIntire papers, FDRL.

Bruenn, a New York City heart specialist, was commissioned in the Navy in 1942 and was assigned to the President. Bruenn was with Mr. Roosevelt when he died. The commander had been with him almost constantly since he was commissioned."[26]

Asked in 1990 about how he came to be assigned to Bethesda Naval Hospital, Bruenn answered, "It was a great mystery to me. I was still in my 30s when I was transferred there ... When I came back after the war I tried to find out how the Navy had obtained information about me. How I got transferred from a ward officer in a boot camp to the head of the cardiology department is still a mystery."[27]

The explanation behind this "mystery" is obvious. Bruenn was recruited because he was at the top of his profession, just as Les Heiter in 1930 and Ross McIntire had been in 1933. Rather than the "young doctor" he is universally portrayed as, Bruenn was one of America's preeminent cardiologists at the time. In late 1942, he was thirty-seven years old, married with a young child and another on the way. He had graduated from Columbia University in 1925, Johns Hopkins Medical School in 1929, and had attained the prestigious title of Professor of Medicine at the College of Physicians and Surgeons at Columbia University School of Medicine.

Bruenn was commissioned Lieutenant Commander in the Navy on November 18, 1942, and began active duty on December 28.[28] After being acclimated to the military while performing physical exams on recruits at the U.S. Naval Training Station in Sampson, New York, he was assigned by Ross McIntire to Bethesda Naval Hospital and reported for duty on April 25, 1943, to serve as "cardiologist for the hospital and consultant to the Third Naval District."[29] This is when Bruenn began treating Franklin. A month later, he also performed a physical examination and an EKG on Eleanor.[30]

"Clinical Notes" provides a cursory review of Franklin's medical history. After discussing Franklin's paralysis from polio in 1921, Bruenn briefly mentions the medical crisis of May 1941 from gastrointestinal bleeding,

26 *Chicago Tribune*, April 13, 1945.
27 Jan Herman interview with Howard Bruenn.
28 Official Military File of Howard Gerald Bruenn, National Archives. https://catalog. archives.gov/id/145767090.
29 *Ibid.*
30 Howard Bruenn papers, FDRL.

parroting the diagnosis Ross McIntire confabulated in his 1951 *U.S. News & World Report* interview. "There was a history in the chart of the development of severe iron deficiency anemia in May 1941, with a hemoglobin of 4.5g/100 ml," Bruenn wrote. "This was apparently due to bleeding hemorrhoids, and the anemia responded quickly to ferrous sulfate [iron] therapy." The blood loss McIntire had characterized in 1951 as "mild" was upgraded to "severe," but the life-saving transfusions Franklin received to treat it were purposely omitted.[31]

The medical events after Franklin's return from Tehran were described. "During the latter part of December 1943, he had an attack of influenza with the usual signs and symptoms—fever, cough, and malaise [feeling badly]. After this he failed to regain his usual vigor and subsequently had several episodes of what appeared to be upper respiratory infections." Surprisingly, Bruenn added "there had been occasional bouts of abdominal distress and distention, accompanied by profuse perspiration." This possibly refers to the event in Tehran described by Charles Bohlen. The plural "bouts" suggest other such episodes may have occurred as well.

At this point "Clinical Notes" devolves into complete fiction. As the false narrative goes, Ross McIntire agreed to have Franklin examined at the naval hospital on Tuesday, March 27, 1944, at the insistence of Anna (actually March 28 according to FDR's daily calendar). Supposedly never having examined Franklin before, Bruenn claims to have made a "wholly unsuspected" diagnosis of severe congestive heart failure and then had to convince a panel of physicians including two "honorary consultants," Doctors James Paullin and Frank Lahey, to permit him to treat Franklin with digitalis. Jim Bishop's 1979 tome about the last year of FDR's life,[32] lays out the bogus story in detail, using, of course, information fed to him by Bruenn. The doctor neglected to tell Bishop about the necessity since at least February 1944 to prop up Franklin's upper body with two by fours or the use of a special bed to relieve his shortness of breath when lying flat.[33] This phenomenon, known as orthopnea, is a classic sign of severe heart failure.[34]

---

31 *Ibid.*
32 Bishop, J., *FDR's Last Year April 1944–April 1945.* New York: William Morrow & Company, 1974, 11–12.
33 To be specific, a "Gatch bed."
34 When the heart's left ventricle fails to adequately pump blood to the body, fluid backs up into the lungs, causing shortness of breath. The heart's burden is reduced when sitting up. This is why two by fours and a Gatch bed were used.

The lies came hard and fast during Bruenn's interview with historian Doris Kearns Goodwin for her 1994 Pulitzer Prize-winning Roosevelt biography, *No Ordinary Time*, another Pulitzer Prize-winning effort. "McIntire was appalled at my suggestions," Bruenn told Goodwin. "The president can't take time off to go to bed," McIntire insisted. "You can't simply say to him do this or do that. This is the president of the United States!" This conversation never happened. For Bruenn to have told the truth—that he had been treating the president since April 1943—would have been to acknowledge a medical condition Franklin supposedly didn't have until a year later.[35]

"One week before being seen," the false narrative continues, "he had developed an acute coryza [an upper respiratory infection] which was followed two days later by an annoying cough with production of small amounts of thick, tenacious, yellowish sputum," Bruenn wrote. Aside from cardiac findings, the paper includes a March 29 urinalysis which Bruenn doctored to remove evidence of a severe urinary tract infection. When bacterial infection strikes the kidney, the body mobilizes white blood cells (pus cells) to fight it. As large amounts of pus cells accumulate, they form casts molded in the shape of the kidney tubules. The presence of casts of pus in the urine is indicative of severe infection. In this case Bruenn selectively excluded mention of "fairly

---

35 Goodwin, D.K., *No Ordinary Time. Franklin and Eleanor Roosevelt: The Home Front in World War II*. New York: Simon & Schuster, 1994. A long fictional narrative of the exam is laid out in detail beginning on page 493. This was probably Bruenn's last interview, marking the end of the postmortem cover-up. Bruenn, 90, died in 1995.

numerous" casts of pus and "mucus strands some enmeshed with pus cells."
His unpublished notes also indicate this condition may have been present
for as long as three years, perhaps as far back as the urinary catheterization
during the "swamp fever" episode in March 1940.

The original laboratory report[36]:

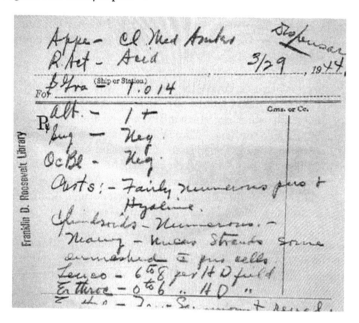

As published[37]:

tion could be held); and urine: specific gravity,
1.014; sugar, 0; albumin, 1 +; numerous hyaline
casts; WBC, 6 to 8 per high power field (hpf); RBC,
0 to 6/hpf.

36 Bruenn Papers, FDRL.
37 "Clinical Notes," 569.

Nowhere in "Clinical Notes" is there any mention of infection, the prostate gland, or the use of antibiotics.

Franklin actually did go to Bethesda in the afternoon of Tuesday, March 28, after spending a weekend at Hyde Park and a day in Washington in his sickbed, where he was almost undoubtedly treated by Bruenn.[38] That date likely marked the time that the cardiologist was necessary on a daily basis and could no longer be hidden from White House staff. His presence remained secret from the press. Bruenn's credentials are not found in otherwise comprehensive Secret Service White House ID files.

Bruenn stated he began a course of treatment with digitalis on April 2, 1944. This canard is destroyed by Dr. George Webster's 1979 letter to Dr. Harry Goldsmith, which reveals that Bruenn saw Franklin on February 2, 1944, and administered the drug. "Clinical Notes" states a decision was made on April 3, 1944, that the president needed "a period of rest and relaxation away from Washington"—the supposed genesis of his four-week stay in South Carolina. The time line clashes with fact. Franklin's February 20 communiqué to Churchill confirms the trip already had been decided upon two weeks before Bruenn was supposed to have first examined him.

Exactly what drugs Franklin was given is unknown. Three effective anti-bacterial agents were available during Franklin's lifetime—none of them were admitted to having been used. The first effective anti-bacterial drug, Sulfadiazine, became popular in America in 1937 after *The New York Times* reported that the newly developed compound had cured FDR Jr. of a potentially fatal throat infection.[39] The Suckley diary documents Franklin Sr. being treated with "sulpha" in January 1943.

Penicillin was developed in the early 1940s and was in widespread use in the military by D-Day. Treatment with Penicillin is sometimes complicated by an itchy skin rash. Franklin complained to labor adviser Anna Rosenberg in 1945 that his "penicillin rash" was keeping him awake.[40] Mortician Hayden Snoderly described Franklin's corpse to be "covered with blisters," an allergic reaction to the drug.[41] Another "miracle drug," streptomycin—first administered to a human at the Mayo Clinic in November 1944—was probably given

---

38 FDR Day by Day, March 28, 1944.
39 "Young Roosevelt Saved by New Drug," *New York Times*, December 17, 1936.
40 Gunther, J., *Roosevelt in Retrospect*. New York: Harper & Brothers, 1950, 365.
41 Snoderly, F.H., *Handwritten Memoir of Franklin Roosevelt's Autopsy*, private collection.

to Franklin at Warm Springs in December, and was a likely cause of his hearing loss that became evident in March 1945.[42]

Ross McIntire never acknowledged giving Franklin any opiate painkiller, though Howard Bruenn admitted to administering codeine, a less potent form of morphine, during Franklin's May 1944 attack of abdominal pain and again at Yalta as a cough suppressant. Harry Goldsmith reported a visit to Havana by one of Franklin's medical aides, almost surely George Fox, who, after drinking heavily, tearfully exclaimed to companions that "FDR had cancer of the prostate which had spread and it was causing him pain to the point where morphine was no longer helping."[43] Exactly when Franklin resorted to using alcohol as a painkiller is unknown, but his son James wrote of his use of it in January 1945 at his fourth inauguration.

Bruenn told Jan Herman in 1990 that Franklin had little interest in his health—a ludicrous assertion to anyone familiar with his involvement in the treatment of his polio.

Herman: "Jim Bishop, in his book, *FDR's Last Year*, over and over says the President didn't ask about his health, and therefore Dr. McIntire didn't tell him. But didn't Roosevelt know how ill he was?"

"He never asked me a question about the medications I was giving him, what his blood pressure was, nothing," Bruenn replied. "He was not interested. He had a job to do and the hell with everything else." Bruenn had been Bishop's source. He also had editorial control *F.D.R.: The Last Year*, a 1980 TV biopic produced by HBO adapted from Bishop's book.[44]

When the Navy medical historian brought up the subject of Frank Lahey, Bruenn came up with a series of whoppers.

> "Lahey, at the only meeting we had following my initial examination [allegedly in April 1944] said, 'This is nothing in my field.' and signed himself off."
>
> Herman: "Lahey really didn't have anything to do with the President's care after that?"

---

42 Lomazow, S., "Was Franklin Delano Roosevelt Treated with Streptomycin?" *Journal of Medical Biography* February 18, 2010;18(1):61.
43 Goldsmith, 142.
44 Jason Robards played the role of Franklin. Eileen Heckert was cast as Eleanor.

Bruenn: "Oh, no, not a bit. To my knowledge, he never saw him again."[45]

Bruenn had written in "Clinical Notes" that "Dr. Lahey was particularly interested in the gastrointestinal tract but submitted that no surgical procedure was needed. He did, however, indicate that the situation was serious enough to warrant acquainting the President with the full facts of the case in order to assure his full cooperation."

Another easily disproved fabrication is the explanation for Franklin's weight loss. "With the low-fat diet that had been enforced since May and the restrictions of calories, there had been a progressive loss of weight of which the President was rather proud and was insistent on a further loss to around 170 lb.," Bruenn wrote. "Despite the best efforts of the cook, liberalization of calories and much persuasion, he obstinately kept himself on his restricted diet."[46] Bruenn echoed Ross McIntire's oft-repeated story that Franklin wanted to lose weight because he was "proud of his flat tummy." Even with the president underweight at 168 pounds in September 1944, Bruenn wrote, "[Franklin] was insistent in his desire to lose more weight."

Daisy Suckley's diary entry on June 27, 1944, shatters that claim. "The P. was weighed today & has gone down to 174 ¾ … He wants to go up a lb. or two, to not be less than 175 & not more than 180. He feels better thin, however, and walked much more easily in the water than a month ago."

Toward the end, Franklin's emaciated appearance aroused profound concern—including his own. On March 12, 1945, Robert Murphy, one of Franklin's most trusted foreign policy advisers, was summoned to update him on the deteriorating situation in Poland. "He was aware of how badly he looked and mentioned he had lost thirty-six pounds," Murphy wrote.[47] The math translates to a shocking 152 pounds. By April 12 he had lost even more, weighing at death between 145 and 150. "Cardiac cachexia," a poorly understood weight loss in patients with severe heart failure, might offer an explanation, but in that condition such a pronounced amount is rarely seen. By far the best explanation for losing forty pounds in sixteen months is cancer.

45 Bruenn interview with Jan Herman.
46 "Clinical Notes," 581.
47 Barach, A.A., "Franklin Roosevelt's Illness: Effect on Course of History." *New York State Journal of Medicine*, 1977;77(13):2154.

"The time from the middle of May to the early part of August was without incident relative to the President's health," Bruenn wrote. "The two days spent in San Diego were busy ones ... The President showed no evidence of fatigue and was intensely interested in the various aspects of the military installations." The excruciating abdominal pain that struck him in his railway car was not mentioned.

Brief, intense spasmodic abdominal pain has many possible causes. One is intussusception, an extraordinarily painful phenomenon in which the bowel suddenly telescopes into itself. Intussusception is uncommon but is known to occur in patients in whom melanoma has metastasized to the small intestine.

Of Franklin's trip to Hawaii in August 1944, Bruenn wrote, "Throughout this period of hectic activity the President moved without obvious fatigue or difficulty of any kind." Harold Ickes reported hearing "disturbing news" from Tom Corcoran that "FDR's health is not good and he had to break some engagements in Honolulu."[48] Seeing Franklin for the first time in years, General Douglas MacArthur observed that, "physically he was just a shell of the man I had known. It was clearly evident that his days were numbered."[49] MacArthur predicted to his staff that the president would be dead within a year.[50] In Hawaii, Franklin visited wounded servicemen and was wheeled through wards of amputees, stopping to chat and to let them see how he had triumphed over his own disability—and how they could do the same. One man was forced to amputate his own leg to survive. "I understand you are something of a surgeon," Franklin told him. "I'm something of an orthopedist myself."[51]

Despite the intensely painful ordeal Franklin endured at his fourth inaugural address, only a brief, dismissive account of the speech appears in the paper. "He gave [the address] without difficulty, although he used his leg braces for the first time since August." Bruenn wrote. The explanation for Franklin's poor performance during his "Yalta speech" to Congress inadvertently confirmed Franklin's visual problem. "He laughingly reported that while giving the speech he had spoken at intervals from memory and 'off the record' and that he had then had slight difficulty in finding the proper place when returning to read the printed words of his address."

---

48 *Ickes Diary*, August 6, 1944. Unpublished, microfilm at FDRL.
49 Wills, M.B., *FDR in 1944: A Diminished President*. Raleigh, NC: Ivy House, 2003, 29.
50 MacArthur, D., *Reminiscences*. Annapolis, MD: Naval Institute Press, 2012, 199.
51 Gallagher, 172–173.

The last paragraph of "Clinical Notes" was written entirely by the Halsteds and reprises one of the paper's primary premises. "I have often wondered what turn the subsequent course of history might have taken if the modern methods for the control of hypertension had been available," the Halsteds wrote in Bruenn's voice.[52]

Another integral part of the Bruenn/Halsted conspiracy was to discredit the competence of Ross McIntire, whose skills as a physician Dr. Halsted had crowed about five years earlier. Anna created this myth in 1967, telling Bernard Asbell, "I didn't think McIntire was an internist who really knew what he was talking about. I felt Father needed more care."[53] Bruenn reiterated the lie to Jan Herman in 1990. "The initial thing that brought me into the picture was Anna," he said. "She put the pressure on Ross McIntire to find out what was going on, because the President was not himself."

The strategy succeeded. After 1970, McIntire was almost universally described as incompetent. Historian Thomas Fleming went so far as to call him a "medical ignoramus."[54] The first attempt to resurrect McIntire's undeserved reputation was this author's paper "Vice Admiral Ross T. McIntire: A Reassessment of an American Hero," published in *Navy Medicine* in 2008.[55]

McIntire's intense devotion to Franklin did not go unrecognized during his lifetime. Frank Lahey, a man not easily given to compliments, wrote in January 1945, "I do not flatter [McIntire] in the least when I say I have never known a more completely unselfish individual in such a high and influential position. He wants nothing for himself. Everywhere I go in the Navy, I talk with commanding officers and they all feel as I do, that the Navy and the country is blessed with such a surgeon general."[56]

Nor did McIntire's self-sacrifice escape the notice of President Truman, who spoke at a luncheon honoring the admiral at Washington's Carlton Hotel on October 30, 1951. "Admiral McIntire is in that category of people that were in the military service when I came to the White House who has been willing to do anything that is necessary for the welfare of the country, and anything that

52 Halsteds to Bruenn, Bruenn papers, FDRL.
53 Asbell, *Mother and Daughter*, 177.
54 Fleming, T., *The War Within World War II*. New York: Basic Books, 2001, 39.
55 Lomazow, S., "Vice Admiral Ross T. McIntire: A Reassessment of an American Hero." *Navy Medicine*, July 2008.
56 Lahey to Albert Q. Maisel, January 29, 1945. Ross McIntire papers, FDRL.

the President has ever asked him to do," Truman said. "It is one of the great satisfactions of being in the office that I occupy that there are people who put the welfare of the Nation above their own personal interests."[57]

57 Truman, H.S. "Remarks at a Luncheon for Vice Admiral Ross T. McIntire," October 30, 1951. Online by Peters, G., Woolley, J.T., *The American Presidency Project*, https://www.presidency.ucsb.edu/documents/remarks-luncheon-for-vice-admiral-ross-t-mcintire; http://www.presidency.ucsb.edu/ws/?pid=13978.

■ Chapter 31
■ Restoring the Truth

"Clinical Notes" was universally accepted as fact. The review in *The New York Times* was published under the headline "Roosevelt's Doctor Says Last Illness Did Not Prevent President From Performing Duties." Virtually every subsequent Roosevelt biographer has heaped praise upon Bruenn for his "truthfulness about Roosevelt's precarious state of health."[1]

By 1970, the dire consequences of severe hypertension had become a well-established fact, so the idea that Franklin had died from that condition was an easy sell. A statistical analysis of Franklin's cardiovascular prognosis by Dr. Hugh Evans in his 2005 book, *The Hidden Campaign: FDR's Health and the 1944 Election*, predicted a life expectancy of less than two years.[2] Evans was correct, as was Bruenn's cardiac prognosis in the Lahey memorandum. Severe hypertension and heart failure would almost surely have killed Franklin prior to 1948—had he not first succumbed to a brain hemorrhage from metastatic melanoma.[3] Considering the sequence of events—well-documented treatment by cancer specialists in the early 1930s, progression and surgical cosmetic erasure of an obviously malignant pigmented lesion, and a left-side visual deficit on March 1, 1945 followed six weeks later by a catastrophic right-sided cerebral hemorrhage—melanoma is a far more probable explanation.

End-stage melanoma metastasizes widely. It has the highest propensity of all cancers to metastasize to the brain. A retrospective study of melanoma patients at Memorial Sloan Kettering Cancer Center (MSKCC) between 1973 and 1976 revealed that one-third had died of central nervous system involvement, most commonly cerebral hemorrhage.[4] Another peer-reviewed paper

---

1 Wills, 155.
2 Evans, 68.
3 The etiology of FDR's malignant hypertension that took hold in 1944 is also a matter for discussion. For instance, and in this case admittedly speculative, his well-documented history of long-standing proteinuria followed by mild then malignant hypertension, fits the profile of a condition that had not yet been described in Roosevelt's lifetime—radiation nephropathy attributable to his treatment for prostate cancer. See: https://core.ac.uk/download/pdf/359176982.pdf.
4 This does not literally mean the primary tumor was in the stomach as was the case with Harry Hopkins, but rather refers to metastatic lesions to the liver and other abdominal or-

in 2009 stated, "Brain metastasis is common in patients with malignant melanoma and represents a significant cause of morbidity and mortality. Nearly 37 percent of patients diagnosed with malignant melanoma eventually develop symptomatic brain metastasis. 75 percent of those who died of the disease had brain metastasis at autopsy."[5] Another autopsy series of melanoma patients conducted at MSKCC revealed that over 75 percent had liver metastases.[6]

In December 1979, Dr. Harry S. Goldsmith published "Unanswered Mysteries in the Health of Franklin D. Roosevelt," in the respected journal *Surgery Gynecology and Obstetrics (SG&O)*,[7] rekindling the conversation about Franklin's melanoma. "Dr. Goldsmith said he was pursuing the possibility of an unrevealed cancer because of the persistence of a rumor that Roosevelt had cancer," *The New York Times* wrote. "The Dartmouth surgeon said he had written the paper with the aim of bringing into sharper focus the medical events that occurred in the last year of Roosevelt's life."[8]

Goldsmith's interest had been piqued by a lecture he attended during his training at MSKCC in the early 1960s, in which iconic cancer surgeon George T. Pack told his audience that his friend, Boston surgeon Frank H. Lahey, had diagnosed Franklin with advanced stomach cancer in 1944. Dr. Lahey had informed the president of the diagnosis, said Pack, and advised

---

gans common in both terminal melanoma and prostatic cancer. See: Ma, B., Wells A.,Wei, L, Zheng, J., "Prostate Cancer Liver Metastasis: Dormancy and Resistance to Therapy." *Review Seminars in Cancer Biology* 2021 June;71:2–9.

"Liver metastasis causes nearly half of death from solid tumors. Metastatic lesions, to the liver in particular, can become detectable years or decades after primary tumor removal, leaving an uncertain long-term prognosis in patients. Prostate cancer (PCa), a prominent metastatic dormant cancer, has the worst prognosis when found in the liver compared to other metastatic sites." The statistics for metastatic melanoma are also dire: "Studies have shown that melanoma can spread to almost any area of the body—a wider variety of areas than any other cancer. The likelihood that it will spread to each organ is as follows: Lymph Nodes: 50% to 75%. Lungs and area between the lungs: 70% to 87%. Liver: 54% to 77%. Brain: 36% to 54%. Bone: 23% to 49%." https://www.verywellhealth.com/where-and-why-can-melanoma-spread-3010811.

5 Barnholtz-Sloan, J.S., Nock, C.J., Einstein, D.B., "Diagnosis and Treatment of Melanoma Brain Metastasis: A Literature Review." *Cancer Control* 2009;16:248–255.

6 Gupta, T.K., Brasfield, R.D., "Metastatic Melanoma of the Gastrointestinal Tract." *Archives of Surgery* 1964;88(6):969–973.

7 Goldsmith, H.S., "Unanswered Mysteries in the Death of Franklin D. Roosevelt." *Surgery, Gynecology, & Obstetrics.* 1979;149:899–908.

8 Altman, L.K., "Surgeon Asserts Roosevelt May Have Had Cancer Before 4th Term." *New York Times*, December 2, 1979, 46.

Franklin that he not run for a fourth term because, in Lahey's opinion, he would not survive that term.

Bruenn fired off an angry response to the editor of *SG&O*, Dr. Loyal Davis.[9] "It was my intention when I wrote my paper in 1970 to set at rest, finally and clearly, all rumors and suspicions about the medical history of President Roosevelt," he wrote on January 18, 1980. "Apparently I failed."

Bruenn lambasted Goldsmith's paper as "so charged with innuendoes, assumptions, inaccuracies, and pure guesses, that it would be futile for me to answer these in detail ... It is ironic that despite Dr. Goldsmith's somewhat frantic search for evidence in this case. He never bothered to get in touch with me. I only happened to be the physician in charge." This argument is similar to what Ross McIntire told the *Washington Times* in 1949 in his effort to discredit Dr. Karl Wold. He told Davis, as he would later tell Jan Herman, that Dr. Lahey had seen President Roosevelt only once, "some two weeks"—actually, four days if one were to believe his false narrative—after he first examined Franklin. "After presenting the clinical and laboratory data which I had assembled, Dr. Lahey's remark was 'There is no problem here for a surgeon.' If Dr. Lahey had suspected a malignancy, it seems to me he certainly would have informed me, inasmuch as I was literally and practically in charge of the case. He made no such remark. At no time was the question of a malignancy suggested to me or to the President."[10]

In 1987, investigative reporter Jack Anderson wrote about a letter he had received from a doctor who had said the same thing as Goldsmith. "Our report rang a bell with Dr. Samuel Day of Jacksonville Florida. Dr. Day, the former president of the Florida Medical Association, recalled a visit in the late 1950s by an old friend and internationally known cancer surgeon, Dr. George Pack. [Pack] related a story which had been told to him by Dr. Frank Lahey," Day wrote. "It seems that President Roosevelt and his entourage came to Boston by special train to see Dr. Lahey prior to his final race for reelection in 1944. After intensive studies at the Lahey Clinic it was found that he had advanced cancer of the stomach ... I am sure that was the stated site, as I was surprised at never having heard of any of FDR's 'stomach ailments' before that.[11] "Dr. Lahey told Dr. Pack that he related

---

9 Davis was the father-in-law of Ronald Reagan.
10 Goldsmith, 73.
11 The cancer was not primary in the GI Tract but metastatic. Numerous anecdotal reports suggest the diagnosis was liver metastases, a very common site of spread from both

the findings to the president and told him he was a very sick man and he could not advise him to run for office again. Mr. Roosevelt was said to have replied, 'Well, I am running,' to which Dr. Lahey replied, 'Well, Mr. President, I would suggest that you take on a strong vice president.' It was apparently understood that this was top-secret information and nothing was published detrimental to the president."

Pack revisited Florida in 1965 and Day asked him whether he had heard anything more about the FDR incident. Pack told him, "I spoke to Dick Cattell [Lahey's successor as head of the Clinic],[12] and he seemed upset by my inquiry. Cattell was quite short with me, saying that was confidential information and will not be released ... [Pack] argued that since both FDR and Lahey were then dead, the information should be released ... Cattell angrily dismissed the subject."[13]

Public Affairs published *FDR's Deadly Secret* in 2010, co-authored by this author and journalist Eric Fettmann. The book revealed details of Franklin's 1941 anemia, exposed his neurological disease, and his death from melanoma. The book received wide press coverage and largely favorable reviews, but, in the end, made little headway toward debunking the well-entrenched myths created by Howard Bruenn and the Halsteds.

The criticism leveled most often at *FDR's Deadly Secret* is the absence of autopsy-based evidence—but this is precisely what Ross McIntire and Franklin himself, as early as 1937, wanted to assure. The only absolute proof of FDR's diagnoses will rest forever in a sealed casket in Sara Delano Roosevelt's rose garden.

As medical science progresses, more scientific evidence supportive of the conclusions in *FDR Unmasked* piles up. In 2018, for instance, Australian researchers found that melanoma patients have a 25 percent greater risk of developing prostate cancer.[14]

---

melanoma and prostate cancer.

12 Cattell was particularly well known for his expertise in gall bladder surgery. It was he who repaired, in Boston, Anthony Eden's lacerated bile duct.

13 "Evidence FDR Knew of Cancer" Jack Anderson and Joseph Spear, *Washington Post*, July 2, 1987.

14 Cole-Clark, D., Nair-Shalliker, V., Bang, A. et al. "An Initial Melanoma Diagnosis May Increase the Subsequent Risk of Prostate Cancer: Results from the New South Wales Cancer Registry." *Scientific Reports* 2018;8:7167.

The story in *FDR Unmasked* does not diminish FDR's accomplishments—it enhances them. It has been nearly eighty years since Franklin's death, and more than a half a century since the Halsteds and Howard Bruenn rewrote history. The intent of this book is to correct the record so historians might remember Franklin Delano Roosevelt as he deserves to be—a man who overcame serious physical challenges at every stage of his political career to become the greatest American president of the twentieth century.

■ INDEX

Teaches Eleanor how to speak in
   public 50,51
Warns Franklin his political career is
   over if he stays with Lucy 33
Howland, Rebecca 2
Hubbard, Dr. Leroy 56
Huggins, Dr. Charles 147
Hughes, Charles Evans 82
Hull, Cordell 127,227
Hull, Lyttle 102
Hurley, Patrick 213,214

Ibn Saud, King of Saudi Arabia 217,219
Ickes, Harold 108,117,122,136,264
Ickes, Jane 117
International Brotherhood of
   Teamsters 186

Jackson, Dr. John Hughlings 197
Jackson, Robert, H. 108
Jackson, Graham 240,241
Jones, Leroy 48,53
Joseph, Louis 53
Josephson, Dr. Emanuel 247

Kaiser, Henry 176
Karig, Walter 121,124,138,141
Kaye, Danny 223
Keen, Dr William W. 43,71,75
Kelly, Edward 126
Kennedy, Dr. Foster 62
Kennedy, John F. 247
Kennedy, Joseph P. 98,113
Kennedy, Rosemary 139n
Kernochan, Frederick 76,77,103
King, Adm. Ernest J. 209
King, Mackenzie 123
Kirklin, Dr. Byrl R. 181
Knowles, Clayton 249
Knox, Alexander 188
Knox, Frank 131,142
Krupp, Friedrich 68
Ku Klux Klan 52

L'Etang, Dr. Hugh 254
LaFollette, Robert 52
LaGuardia, Fiorello 135
Lahey Clinic 195
Lahey Memorandum 173,174
Lahey, Dr. Frank H. 147,149,151,173,
   174,246,252,259,270
Lake, Veronica 195
Lambert, Dr. Samuel 62
Landon, Alfred 107
Lane, Franklin 27
Lansing, Robert 34
Lape, Esther 51
Larooco 50,51
Law, Nigel 30
Lawrence, John 50
League of Nations 34,36
Leahy, Adm. William 137
LeHand, Marguerite "Missy" 36,39,48,
   50–55,58,85,107,115
Levine, Dr. Samuel 43
Liberty magazine 62,63,127,122,125,
   138,141,248
Life Magazine 179,211
Lincoln, Abraham 207
Lindbergh, Charles 142
Lion and the Fox 255
Lipson, Milton 201
Locock, Dr. Charles 197
Lomazow, Dr. Steven 109,266
Long, Breckinridge 180
Longworth, Alice
   Roosevelt 10,15,30,31,33
Longworth, Nicholas 33
Looker, Earl 62,63
Lost Horizon 166
Lovett, Dr. Robert W. 43,46,48
Loyless, Tom 61,62
Lynch, Thomas, E. 18

MacArthur, Gen. Douglas 72,181,
   213,264
Mack, John E. 18
MacLeish, Archibald 206,224
Maloney, Francis 201
Maloney, Helena 56
Malta 209

Wilson, Edith Bolling Galt 29,208,
   233,246
Wilson, Ellen Axson 28
Wilson, Woodrow 28–30,132,138,215
Wold, Dr. Karl C. 155,200,249,252,271
Women's Digest magazine 248,250
Woodin, William 97
Works Progress Administration
   (WPA) 99
Wright, James L. 96

Yalta 174,195,199,208–217,228,263
Young, John Russell 122,125

Zangara, Giuseppe 76,78